The Person-Centered Approach: Applications for Living

The Person-Centered Approach: Applications for Living

Doug Bower

Writers Club Press
San Jose New York Lincoln Shanghai

The Person-Centered Approach: Applications for Living

Writers Club Press
an imprint of iUniverse.com, Inc.

For information address:
iUniverse.com, Inc.
5220 S 16th, Ste. 200
Lincoln, NE 68512
www.iuniverse.com

ISBN: 0-595-14705-4

Printed in the United States of America

Contents

Back to the Very Basic Basics

Dedication

I dedicate this material to the late Theron Nease, Ph.D., whose belief in me set me on a path to higher education, counseling, supervision, and teaching.

Just before I finished my Master of Divinity, T. told me that if I would do a year of Clinical Pastoral Education he would help get me into the Master of Theology program at Columbia Theological Seminary in Decatur, Ga. At that point, I had only dreamed of the possibility of doing formal graduate studies, but I did not believe it was possible for me.

When I successfully completed the C.P.E. program, T. was good to his word. I do not have a clue how he got me into the program. I do know there was opposition to my entering the program.

During that pilgrimage, T. developed cancer and died before I finished the degree. It was a significant lose for me as T. was my mentor and I held him in high esteem.

When I tried to graduate, the opposition that resisted my entrance to the program resisted my graduation. We had a major falling away. I did not get out of that program with a degree. Between my stubbornness and the stubbornness of the folks who had poor regard from my performance, I decided not to get that degree and instead focused on completing my doctoral work.

I also dedicate this material to Jerold Bozarth, Ph.D., who was first my mentor and teacher, and now my colleague in the Person-Centered Approach to education, counseling, and supervision.

It was Jerold's introductory course to the theories and practice of counseling and psychotherapy, and his commitment to the Person-Centered Approach to counseling and psychotherapy that gave me the first solid glimpses of the theory I know use as the basis of my work in counseling, teaching, ministry, writing, editing, and what little nursing I still do.

We have worked together on a number of projects including the Person-Centered Journal, and the annual Warm Springs Workshop. We have fussed with each other, and laughed with each other. I wouldn't be person-centered without his participation in my pilgrimage. Since I was scrambling at the time I met in 1982, I don't know what I would be as a theorists. Of the approaches I have investigated, cct/pca makes the most sense, though I am also quick to say there is aspects of the theory that are nonsense to me.

Jerold didn't produce a cct/pca robot. I suspect at times to his delight and at other times to his dismay. He did help produce a person loyal to the Person-Centered Approach, skeptical and critical of it at times, and a staunch defender of it at other times. I can say with confidence, I have developed an international reputation in the approach. This is exciting to me as a person who hardly felt noticed in his own high school in the 60s.

I have been touched and dismayed by the people in this approach. I again thank T. and Jerold for being a part of my pilgrimage.

Foreword

My mentor and colleague, Jerold Bozarth wrote in the forward for Person-Centred Counselling in Action by Dave Mearns and Brain Thorne, (1988): "It is noteworthy that this is the first comprehensive and systematic text concerning the client-centred approach since Rogers' book, Client-Centered Therapy (1951)."

Over the years, it hadn't occurred to me this was the case. It had occurred to me that the approach was too closely associated with one man, Carl Rogers. It also occurred to me that the approach sounded like a broken record, that is the focus has been to rearticulate the "necessary and sufficient conditions" or the "core conditions" again, and again, and again. In some ways it has felt to me as if those of us who espouse this approach have our heads stuck in the apologetics of the approach rather than telling the world what we have seen and heard.

I am pleased to say that recent efforts seem to me to interested in dealing with the theory in relationship to real human issues and applications. This project is such an effort.

There are people with real problems and real struggles. Can this approach to be applied to daily living, to the trauma's of living, to the struggles that people have? My position is yes. However, let us demonstrate the applications.

I feel comfortable that this project has done that. There is theory here. There is also application here.

In the future, I hope to present book projects on community mental health, education, ministry, and sexuality. The topics are endless. The person-centered approach should be in the midst of the human condition. After all that is where people are persons.

Preface

This project is about variety and applications concerning the Person-Centered Approach and is based on the concept introduced by Carl Rogers and his colleagues. We are not seeking simply to augment his theory though but to speak to the theory from various perspectives.

It is not about perfection, or purity, but about real people and real ideas. The material was not written and edited to please readers. Rather, it was written with the simple idea that authors have something to say and readers are perfectly capable of deciding if they find the material valuable, informative, or worth their while to read.

Each article was reviewed and revised based on feedback. However, the reviews and the feedback was not designed to coerce rewrites that were to keep reviewers happy. Further, we made no effort to have things written to keep readers happy either. Reviewers were charged to look for factual errors, in as much as this is possible in this age of differing perspectives on what is fact. They were also charged with readability. I am not interested in producing a project that only a handful of people can understand.

Thus, this project is about having genuine dialogues between authors and readers, rather than an interaction with what reviewers and editors think readers want or like.

Each contributor has assured me that he or she has written the article that he or she is satisfied with. That is, the contributions say what the author wants to say. It is now up to the reader to decide if the material is something he or she is satisfied with.

Acknowledgments

I sought to cut through my presuppositions about editing and reviewing. I wanted a project that would allow the writers to write. To get to this place, I gave contributors two options. They could send their work to me and I could find reviewers, or they could find three reviewers themselves, and I would publish the material as is except for publication style. In this case, I used the 3rd edition of the "Publication Manual of the American Psychological Association."

I am pleased that a number of reviewers added integrity to this project. Some I have had the privilege of meeting over the years and some I have only heard of and some I have only had dialogue with via e-mail.

I want to thank the following people for reviewing material either at my request or the request of the contributors:

Paula Bickham, Eastern Kentucky University
Jerold Bozarth, professor emeritus, University of Georgia
Jo Cohen, Kutztown University
Robert (Bob) Lee, Center for the Studies of the Person
Bruce Meador, Center for the Studies of the Person
Dottie Morgan, Ft. Valley State University
Ken Newton, professor emeritus, University of Tennessee
Jules Seeman, professor emeritus, Vanderbilt University
Suzanne Spector, Center for the Studies of the Person
William Stillwell, Center for the Studies of the Person
Joachim Schwarz, Center for the Studies of the Person
Chuck Stewart, Assumption College
Carol Topping, Southern College of Technology

List of Contributors

Jerold Bozarth: Professor Emeritus, University of Georgia.

Barbara Temaner Brodley: Illinois School of Professional Psychology.

Richard Bryant-Jefferies: Acorn Community Drug and Alcohol Service, Guildford, England.

Jody DeRidder: graduate teaching assistant, University of Tennessee.

Bryan Farha: Director of Graduate Study in Counseling, Oklahoma City University.

Marlene M. Kuskie: University of Nebraska at Kearney.

David Meador: Center for Studies of the Person, LaJolla, CA.

Susan Bonner Schwarz, & Joachim Schwarz: Center for the Studies of the Person, LaJolla, CA.

Elisabeth Zinschitz: private practice, Vienna, Austria.

Introduction

Like everything else in this project, the introduction was written several times. First, I tried to present a summary of each section. Then I tried to make a basic statement about each contribution. I finally decided that offering the reader my perspective violated the intent of this project, to let author and reader communicate with the minimum of interference.

Certainly part of my decision to not summarize the contents of each chapter was my own sense of futility to doing so as well as my own sense of inadequacy at doing so. The futility and adequacy was not related to feeling I could share my understanding of what has been written, but the sense that I could not do justice to the writer, including my own writing.

Writers and readers have vast resources for interacting with each other whether there is understanding or not. I see no reason to impose myself on that process by getting authors to conform to my expectations, or those of reviewers. Writers are quite capable of deciding if their efforts say what they want them to say. The readers are quite capable of deciding whether they like the materials or not, or agree with them or not.

I am also pleased to submit the project in the relatively new domain of "On-Demand Publishing" via the Internet. While it is possible that this form of publishing will not catch-on, I like the risk involved. I like the freedom to publish that is available. The form is perfect for this project. I am free to publish this project with the philosophy I have in mind. I don't have to keep editors or publishers happy. I don't even have to keep readers happy.

This is a wonderful time to publish and share ideas.

In this I am pleased to submit this project to you the reader for your consideration. Readers may find awkwardness, or wonderment, or annoyance, of excitement in these pages. I don't know what readers' experiences will be.

I now entrust this project to the readers. I am convinced that if readers like what they see, they will either ask for more or venture into this arena themselves.

By the way, the reader will not some apparent spelling discrepancies. For instance, person-centered may be spelled person-centred. This is because of the contributions from outside the U.S. I am pleased to see that participation in this project. I have left those differences intact.

Where We Came From

An E-mail Interaction with Nat Raskin

Doug Bower

It took me some time to engage the Internet, but I finally broke down and purchased a 2400 baud modem. I am now using a 56000 baud modem. Shortly after my first purchase I joined the person-centered e-mail network. As interaction came across that network, I thought it might be unique and valuable to try to conduct an e-mail interview via that media. I approached Nat Raskin, professor emeritus at Northwestern University, whom I met originally at the first annual Warm Springs Conference in 1987. He agreed to participate. Nat Raskin studied with Carl Rogers at Ohio State. He has been a significant part of the client-centered/person-centered approach to therapy and education.

This interaction and the following preparation of the material took over a year to put together. Conflicts in schedules, difficulty in determining a format, and other responsibilities of the interviewer kept the material from being ready sooner. The use of the Internet and e-mail has skyrocketed, yet I have seen no interview conducted via this media. It is therefore still on the cutting edge. I wanted to try to preserve the nature of the interaction as it appeared via the e-mail format. Unfortunately, that format doesn't lend itself to the journal format. I have had to alter the presentation of the material accordingly. However, I didn't altar the content of the questions or responses. Please forgive the awkwardness of the representation of the format.

Opening E-mail Communication to Nat Raskin

I believe we are about to embark on a new pilgrimage together. E-mail is very new to me. Its technology isn't. I have been using telephones, and computers for several years. However, it is new to me to put these together.

We are on the cutting edge of technology, as you pointed on in an e-mail communication over the pca network recently, Bill Gates of Microsoft has been pushing this technology as have a host of others.

When I began to prepare this interaction, a news report stated that Gates and McCaw Cellular Communications were preparing to establish the Teledisc Corporation which would be a major satellite communication network designed to handle phone calls and high resolutions images. So much has happened though that I don't know anything about the status of that endeavor. I only know that I was impressed by the optimism of the project. The Internet is reportedly growing by 1 million new members every month. This news in the world of the Internet is very old news.

I have no idea what direction this E-Mail interview will take. I have a series of questions to ask of you. However, I do not know if we will get to all of them. I have no idea what questions might emerge as a result of this interaction we are having. It seems to me that therapy is the same. I do not know what direction my client and I will take. I try to be open to all sorts of directions.

It also occurred to me that traditionally an interview focuses upon the interviewee. Perhaps you might have statements or questions to address to me as we go.

Question 1

1. Please describe the circumstances under which you met Carl Rogers and share your initial impression of him. Had you heard of him before you met him and under what circumstances did you recall hearing about him.

Answer to Question 1

I was in my senior year at the College of the City of New York in 1940 and was looking into graduate programs in Clinical Psychology. We had a new Department of Psychology chair, the eminent Gardner Murphy. He told me about a new young professor at Ohio State University, Carl Rogers, who had been hired to replace Professor Goddard, known for his work on mental retardation and the Goddard Form Board, a non-verbal, performance measure of intelligence.

I had applied to three other graduate programs in the Midwest: Indiana University, Iowa State, and the University of Minnesota. Each of these had a clinical psychology program headed by a well-known person. But I wrote to Dr. Rogers, received an encouraging reply, applied to Ohio State (even though I came from a not-well-off immigrant family, I was able to afford the tuition—$75 a quarter for out-of-state residents) and with a few other brave souls from City College, made the big change from New York City to Columbus, Ohio.

Even though I was going from a big city to what felt like a small town, it was quite an adventure. I was only 19, living with a roommate in a private home off the campus, had all my meals out, a new experience, and met students from Ohio and other states around the country. Another aspect of the cultural change was moving from the Bronx and New York with a large Jewish population to an environment where Jews were a tiny minority. I was to encounter some institutional anti-Semitism, but felt no barrier in becoming friends with my fellow and sister graduate students; I was excited by the differences.

Carl in person was very welcoming. He seemed like a nice mild-mannered person, easy to talk to, not at all forbidding or charismatic. He was a really good teacher, extremely popular with the new graduate student population, unpopular with some of his peers in the Psychology Department, which might have been the largest in the United States at the time.

Carl seemed very different from the other psychologists on the faculty. Many of them were nationally known, but I found them disappointing in the flesh. Carl stood out for his genuineness, his genuine liking for students, and interest in being associated with them. He had us to his new home, and we met his wife and his two children, who were attending the University School. This was also a wonderful new experience, very different from what I had known in New York.

Doug, I have to stop for now. I'll resume later today or tomorrow morning. Let me know if you're getting what you want, or whatever.

Question 1 a

1 a. You stated that Carl Rogers was a "really good teacher" and he "seemed very different from the other psychologists on the faculty." You mentioned that he stood out for his "genuineness," and "his genuine liking for students." Part of my dissertation (Bower, 1989) was based on the premise that if therapists are transparent, all sorts of attributes or characteristics would be noted. What other characteristics did you note of Carl Rogers that made him a "really good teacher," and seem "very different?" What other characteristics did you note as his student? And what other characteristics did you note through the years?

Answer to Question 1 a

At that point in time (Ohio State University, 1940-42), I meant by "a really good teacher":

(1) that Carl was very clear and logical in his own thinking and communicated his ideas very clearly,

(2) that he gave his students "hands-on" experience in interviewing, counseling undergraduate students, working with mothers and "problem children," etc., and thereby showed great confidence and trust in us (I was only 19 when this started),

(3) the genuineness and genuine liking for us that I've mentioned,

(4) making himself available for individual meetings with us,

(5) being attentive and all there at such meetings, rather than glancing at his watch, or whatever,

(6) inviting us to his home for food, fun and games, with his wife and children.

Later on (at the University of Chicago, 1945-1957), what was added was his conception of himself as a facilitator of learning and fellow-learner rather than a teacher and the accompanying transfer of responsibility to students of specific course content, "assignments," and evaluation.

Still later, in his California years, he became more informal and emotionally and physically free and expressive. Some of this is detailed in his description of his attitudes and behavior in groups in "Carl Rogers on Encounter Groups," (1970).

Question 1 b

1 b. I experience you as humble but assertive. You readily speak-up in the community groups. You have always struck me as warm and kind. Your intelligence is not flaunted and while you speak your mind you don't strike me as overbearing with your ideas and thoughts. What attributes/characteristics do you have that you bring to bear as a educator, therapist?

Answer to Question 1 b

I think what you are picking up is a very strong interest in what others (clients, students, children, members of the community) feel and think combined with seeing myself as an equal in whatever process is going on, rather than falling back on having more power as a teacher, therapist, etc.. Part of it is that I don't feel comfortable addressing a group as a lecturer. I feel much better about being an equal member of a group and having my say as one person. In that position, I have developed the courage increasingly to express my thoughts and even my feelings. It's not at all easy, but I can even cry in a group now and accept it, not feel I have to cover my face.

I believe that very slowly, I've developed some self-confidence over the years which has made my group participation easier, made it possible for me to ask for things to which I feel entitled, and express my anger on the spot when I feel that I am being mistreated. I grew up a shy boy, loved but over-protected, not given enough responsibility, and not being provided with a model of fighting for my rights.

Questions 2 a, & b

2. Who were some of your peers at Ohio State that went on to make contributions to the Client-Centered/Person-Centered Approach?

2 a. Are there any recollections concerning any of those peers you can share? Were there others who made contributions to the psychological or counseling literature of other theories?

Answers to Questions 2, & 2a

I am glad you asked about this, because my peers at Ohio State in the early 1940s were truly impressive. Some of them and their contributions follow:

VIRGINIA AXLINE did graduate work at Ohio State with Rogers shortly after I had left there for military service, and I did not meet her until I got to the University of Chicago in 1946. There, she developed a play therapy program at the Counseling Center and wrote the book "Play Therapy," which gave her national recognition. She moved to Teachers College, Columbia University, where she held spellbound classes of several hundred students with accounts of how children in the understanding, respectful, and encouraging atmosphere of the playroom learned the excitement of self-discovery and acceptance.

ARTHUR COMBS, after graduating from Ohio State, became Director of the Counseling Center at Syracuse University in New York State, and met Donald Snygg from nearby Oswego State College. Together they wrote "Individual Behavior," perhaps the most influential psychology book of this century in demonstrating the importance of the phenomeno-logical experience of the perceiving organism (human or other animal) as a determinant of behavior. Combs went on to a pre-eminent position in the application of client-centered principles to counselor education.

BERNARD J. ("Bud") COVNER was a student of Rogers in Rochester, New York and followed him to Ohio State University, where he was indispensable in setting up the technology for making sound recordings of interviews. Bud also documented, in his doctoral dissertation and in four published articles, the inadequacy of notes compared with electronic recording. He became a leading consultant to industry in the application of client-centered principles.

CHARLES A. CURRAN, a Catholic priest, wrote the books, "Personality Factors in Counseling," (1945) and "Counseling and Psychotherapy: The Pursuit of Values" (1968) and became a principal member of the psychology faculty at Loyola University in Chicago.

THOMAS GORDON followed Rogers to Chicago, wrote the chapter in "Client-Centered Therapy" (1951) on "Group-Centered Leadership and Administration," and has become known around the world for his books and courses on Parent Effectiveness Training and Leader Effectiveness Training.

DONALD K. GRUMMON also followed Rogers to the University of Chicago, where he was a counselor, teacher and key member of the Counseling Center administrative team. He took a job at Michigan State University, where he taught and directed the university's Counseling Center for many years.

NICHOLAS HOBBS directed programs at George Peabody College of Vanderbilt University and Teachers College, Columbia University. He wrote an outstanding article in the American Psychologist on the role of insight in psychotherapy and had a major interest in formulating program standards for disadvantaged children. He was elected President of the American Psychological Association in 1966.

E. H. PORTER, Jr.'s Ph.D. dissertation, "The Development and Evaluation of a Measure of Counseling Interview Procedures" (1941), was important enough to be summarized in detail by Rogers in his first therapy book, "Counseling and Psychotherapy," (1942). Categorizing the state-ments in 19 phonographically recorded interviews, Porter unveiled sharp contrasts between directive and nondirective counseling approaches. Porter was one of Rogers' students who followed him to the University of Chicago and was a key person in applying client-centered principles to the training of Veterans Administration counselors at the U. of C. Counseling Center, an experience which, in turn, helped to advance the whole concept of stu-dent-centered learning.

VICTOR ("Vic") RAIMY's doctoral dissertation, "Self-Reference in Counseling Interviews," is cited by Ruth Wylie in her book, "The Self-Concept" (1961) as the first use by a psychologist of the method of coding interviews with respect to expressed attitudes toward the self. Aside from his research contribution, Raimy contributed a comprehensive for-mulation of self-theory. He focused on learnings about the self as the key type of learning in therapy.

Raimy's contribution to client-centered theory was seminal. He went on to a distinguished career in the Department of Psychology at the University of Colorado, and became known for his professional contribu-tions to the training of clinical psychologists, not just client-centered ther-apists. He organized national training conferences at the University of Colorado, out of which grew the "Boulder Model," which spelled out a scientist-practitioner conception of clinical psychology education, which had a lasting influence on doctoral programs. A central figure in the devel-opment of client-centered theory, Raimy came to believe that a more effective approach to therapy was directive, rational, and cognitive.

WILLIAM U. SNYDER also pioneered in research on patterns of counselor and client behavior and edited the "Casebook of Non-Directive Counseling" (1947). Bill first directed a program for many years at Pennsylvania State University, where he published a major study on "The Psychotherapeutic Relationship," after which he became head of coun-selor training at Ohio University in Athens, Ohio. Like Vic Raimy, he came to prefer a rational-cognitive approach to therapy.

BERNARD STEINZOR was one of a handful of students who went to Ohio State from the College of the City of New York as I did in the fall of 1940, and who continued his graduate study with Rogers at the University of Chicago. He often challenged Carl because of his (Steinzor's) belief in the influence of socio-economic factors on behavior. Steinzor later joined the staff of the Menninger Foundation and in the 1980s, supervised clinical work at an institution in Sweden.

I was friendly with and looked up to many of these individuals. They were creative, articulate, and often fun to be around. Most of them had backgrounds very different from mine. The first time I ever got drunk was with Bill Snyder in Columbus, Ohio. "Dr. Rogers" and his wife Helen often invited us to their home. We would usually meet as a group at the annual conventions of the American Psychological Association, sensing that we were part of a movement that was spelling out some new and exciting directions in American psychology.

Axline, Curran, Grummon, Hobbs, Porter, and Raimy are now dead.

Question 2 b

2 b. I wanted to share my reaction to your response to my second question. I just want to say, Wow! While I had not heard of all these folks, I had heard of most of them and read their works. Needless to say I was impressed that you had the opportunity to be associated with these folks. I don't believe I need a response to this unless it somehow triggers additional thoughts.

Answer to Question 2 b

I feel very fortunate to have had such peers, friends, and people to look up to.

Question 3 & 3b

In 1987, the first year that I met you at Warm Springs, Carl Rogers had just died. His memorial services had not even been held at that time. You gave a presentation there on the historical situation into which the client-centered theory emerged. I don't believe those observations have been published though Jerold Bozarth invited students to summarize various presentations for publication in the "Person-Centered Review" (Bozarth 1987). I summarized your presentation.

What was going on historically and/or theoretically that contributed to the development of the client-centered theory. Were there others working on empathy, unconditional regard, and congruence which may have influenced the development of the approach?

3 a. What was going on historically that was in sharp contrast to this new movement?

Your interest in how you present yourself as a "teacher" is one that I struggle with as I find the traditional role of "expert" and "all knowing" professor a very uncomfortable position. Not only do I not like it, I have never been able to move into the arena of being a walking encyclopedia. My mind gets too garbled and somebody always asks me something I don't know and I think I ought to know. Your position on this is very encouraging to me. I like the more equalitarian situation. I have been trying to maintain the attitude of a facilitator in a program on substance abuse that I have contracted for concerning men who have been sentenced to a diversion center for violating their probation, and who have "misused" or "abused" substances. I really haven't found it hard to do so, but I cannot say I feel it is helpful. Patience and "faith" seems to me to be important when I feel uncomfortable about the seeming lack of "progress" or "direction" the participants take.

Answers to Question 3 & 3 a

It is easier to start with the second half of your question. The field of counseling and psychotherapy was dominated by approaches which emphasized guidance and interpretation, and Rogers himself had been trained in such an environment at Teachers College, Columbia University and at the psychoanalytic Institute of Child Guidance in New York City.

He tried it out for most of his twelve years as a child guidance psychologist and agency director in Rochester, New York, then experimented with an approach which he summarized in "Some Newer Concepts of psychotherapy," the title of his talk at the University of Minnesota in December, 1940. This approach included principles such as:

* Therapy is not a matter of doing something to the individual, or of inducing him to do something about himself. It is instead a matter of freeing him for normal growth and development, of removing obstacles so that he can again move forward.
* Emotional or feeling aspects are stressed rather than intellectual elements, and more emphasis is placed upon the individual's immediate situation than upon the past; the therapeutic relationship itself is valued as a growth experience.
* The client's frame of reference is the therapist's basic consideration, rather than his own appraisal of what is going on.

Rogers was stimulated in the direction of such principles by some exposure to the ideas of psychoanalyst Otto Rank and psychologist Jessie Taft who were at the University of Pennsylvania and the Philadelphia Child Guidance Clinic in the 1930s. I examined their relationship to the development of nondirective therapy in an article on that subject in the Journal of Consulting Psychology in 1948. At Rochester Rogers hired a Philadelphia social worker named Elizabeth Davis, who was systematically recognizing and accepting feelings in her work with clients.

But it was Rogers, with the invaluable collaboration of his students, who articulated a systematic system of psychotherapy based on the belief that clients could guide themselves, and who started the electronic recording of interviews and whole cases, leading to a new era of research on psychotherapeutic process and outcome. It took another five years (1945-6) to begin applying the principles to teaching and other aspects of human relations and about ten more (1957) to evolve the triad of therapist-offered conditions.

Question 4

4. In what ways, if any, has the Client-Centered Theory evolved?

Answer to Question 4

This is such a huge question that I will try to answer it only in a very general way. For a more detailed response, I have a chapter called "Person-Centered Psychotherapy: Twenty Historical Steps," coming out in a British book published by Sage, "Developments in Psychotherapy: Historical Perspectives." Windy Dryden (Ed.). Maybe I'll just mention some of those steps pertaining to theory, starting with the publication of Client-Centered Therapy (1951).

The client's struggle was conceptualized as going beyond the search for solutions to problems. It had to do with the struggle to be oneself, and to live one's experience.

Rogers put forward a 19-proposition theory of personality to accompany his theory of therapy.

Rogers saw the growth force in the client as rooted in a drive for order in the universe.

Client-centered principles were applied to the classroom, to the workplace, to administration, to group therapy, and to play therapy, in effect constructing a person-centered approach to areas of human relations outside of counseling and psychotherapy, even though the phrase, "person-centered approach," was not yet being used in 1951.

The therapist was seen as participating as a whole person in the therapeutic relationship.

Growth in the client was seen as going beyond increased self-esteem and involving openness to experience and the willingness to be a process.

Rogers formulated the "necessary and sufficient conditions of therapeutic personality change." (1957)

Rogers (1959) wrote "A Theory of Therapy, Personality, and Interpersonal Relationships, As Developed in the Client-Centered Framework" for Sigmund Koch's Psychology: A Study of a Science.

With his associates, Rogers applied client-centered theory to group experiences and educational reform following his move to California in 1964.

The concepts of person (e.g. the socially oriented and responsible "person of tomorrow") and of community (communities of workshop and conference participants and the growing international community of persons interested in the person-centered approach) have been clarified and strengthened.

Question 5

5. What are the differences, if any, between the Client-Centered and Person-Centered ideologies?

Answer to Question 5

For me, the ideology is the same. The principles of Client-Centered Therapy spread to other aspects of human relations, such as education and conflict resolution, creating the concept of a Person-Centered Approach. I view Client-Centered Therapy as the Person-Centered Approach applied to the field of psychotherapy.

Question 5 a

5 a. In virtually every meeting related to the client-centered/person-centered approach that I have attended there have been charges made that some claim to be person-centered but are not. Material presented in the Person-Centered Review (Bozarth & Brodley, 1986; Cain, 1986) clearly confront this issue. Do you believe that the slant given to Rogers works by some theorists have distorted Rogers theory? If so, how has Rogers theory become distorted. If no, how is the work of Gendlin and others consistent with Rogers?

Answer to Question 5a

I have referred to a recent historical chapter I have written on the person-centered approach. A section of it deals with the issue you raise:

"The introduction by Gendlin, Gordon, Natalie Rogers, and Garry Prouty of systematic direction in their work raises an issue which divides adherents of the person-centered approach. This is true even though the interventions do not force any particular idea, feeling, or action on their students or clients, and even though their purpose is to further some goal which is seen as a desirable outcome of client-centered work, such as heightened awareness, increased empathy, greater creativity, and readiness for therapy. While these innovators believe they are being consistent with client-centered ideology and that they are furthering a person-centered process, other students of the approach are of the opinion that they do violence to basic person-centered tenets. Barbara Brodley, Jerold Bozarth, Tony Merry, Ruth Sanford, John Shlien and others argue with equal conviction that the belief in the client's capacities articulated with great eloquence by Rogers and others rules out intentional and systematic direction. They cannot integrate with their basic assumptions of the person-centered approach strategies of confrontation or the devising of special methods for dealing with clients based on diagnostic or psychopathological assessment."

I wrote further: "The very first historical step articulated in this paper was: 'Therapy is not a matter of doing something to the individual, or of inducing him to do something about himself. It is instead a matter of freeing him for normal growth and development, of removing obstacles so that he can again move forward' (Rogers, 1942, p. 29). While it has also been brought out here that Rogers himself became more free in his behavior as a therapist or group facilitator, this activity did not take the form of systematic direction." These quotes are from the chapter mentioned in my answer to Question 4, in the book, "Developments in Psychotherapy: Historical Perspectives," Windy Dryden (Ed.), to be published by Sage. Please use only with the permission of the author.

I respect the right of Gendlin and the others who try systematically to stimulate some particular kind of client behavior or experience to label their work "client-centered" or "person-centered." But I believe that, in practicing as they do, they are, in your terms, distorting Rogers' theory, which is based on a nondirective premise.

Question 6 & 6 a

6. Clearly the client-centered (nondirective) theory was on the cutting edge or frontier of the development of psychotherapy, counseling, and education. Just as clearly the theory has not enjoyed that reputation in recent years. What directions do client-centered/person-centered theorists need to take to get back into the forefront of discovery and innovation?

6 a. Carl Rogers, Betty Shearer, you and others did not have client-centered literature on which to base your research. It seems to me that many of the articles on the person-centered approach lead one to the same basic articles. Have today's CC/PC researchers gotten too dependent on each other such that the contemporary researcher might be limiting the theory and thus limiting the range of new discoveries? If so, what are your recommendations.

Answers to Question 6 & 6 a

Again I am more impressed by the diversity that exists. The people who are seen as "true believers" differ among themselves and include some very original thinkers, who sometimes make use of sources that are very distant from the "person-centered" literature. An examination of the programs of our national and international conferences or of the contents of our journals brings out the range of opinion and interest.

Question 7

Questions 6, & 7 seem related to me. I do believe they are questions related to articulating the essence of the person-centered approach and what we find and discover about it. I am somewhat reluctant to ask question number 7 because of its repetitious nature. Yet, even in therapy the same theme emerges over and over and therapists have to seek to understand the differing slants to the same issue. I don't believe that I should discourage the process of understanding because I feel slight discomfort or lack of clarity as to that understanding so I submit the following questions anyway.

First, I wanted to respond to your answers for 6a and 6b. It was the first difference we have had in this interview. Your answers seemed very affirming of the status of the client-centered/person-centered approach in the contemporary psychotherapeutic scene. However, I do not believe that client-centered therapy is on the cutting edge and frontier of the development of psychotherapy any longer. I would suggest that cognitive behaviorism, solution-focused, brief therapy, and the family therapies are far more prominent in the contemporary arena.

Further, I am not at all convinced of the "independent thinking and theorizing going on or the "original thinkers." I do agree that they "sometimes make use of sources that are very distant from the 'person-centered' literature."

I recently did a literature search which produced only 547 articles related to client-centered theory. Another search into alcoholism produced over 11,000 articles. Only three of which were related to the client-centered theory (Pfeiffer, Feuerlein, & Brenk-Schulte, 1991; Dana, 1985; Obitz, 1975). Thank goodness for computers because I would have had a heck of time finding these articles. Even in this, all three were comparing different theories in relationship to differing aspects of alcoholism like motivation for treatment, assertiveness, and other dimensions. There did not seem to me to be any investment in client-centered practice or theory in relationship to the issue of alcoholism. Further, with literally thousands of articles on a variety of issues and topics only 547 emerged from my efforts as related to the client-centered theory. That doesn't demonstrate to me much resourcefulness, research, or creativity being brought to bear on the person-centered approach.

In addition, I would point out the demise of the Person-Centered Review which had been published by a major publisher who abandoned it because there was not enough interest in such a journal. The efforts of

ADPCA to produce a journal are very sufficient for the needs of the person-centered community, but we do not have the support of a major publisher to help us reach out to potentially interested persons.

In this I am very concerned about the future of the approach. In a conversation I had with John Shlien in Warm Springs a couple of years ago, he was very concerned about the apparent decline of the approach. I tried to assure him that the Warm Springs workshop remains strong. I am encouraged by the international workshops, the annual meeting of the ADPCA (Association for the Development of the Person-Centered Approach), and especially the Warm Springs conference. However, I see little indication in the circles in which I run that there is much interest in the person-centered approach. At best, the approach is seen as a good place to start with new psychologists, and counselors, but at worse it is often abandoned in favor of other approaches.

Having stepped up on that soap box, I continue with my questions.

Response to "Soap Box"

"I agree that the person-centered approach is not very influential in the contemporary psychotherapeutic scene, in the United States. I believe that the situation is very different in the British Isles and on the European continent, and perhaps in Latin America and Japan. I also see a lot of life in the movement in the United States, and it remains very important theoretically as the only orientation which facilitates a therapeutic process in which the client is the architect.

I am also not surprised by the small number of client-centered references on the subject of alcoholism or other specific problems, because a basic tenet of the approach is that you offer a cluster of therapeutic conditions to a person irrespective of the problem presented, the degree of emotional disturbance, etc.. I recognize there are people like Garry Prouty, Margaret Warner, and David Cain, who see themselves as client-centered but differ with this principle.

Question 7 (Continued)

Barbara Brodley (1994) reported a portion of an interview in which Carl Rogers wondered if he had spent too much writing time on the "necessary and sufficient conditions" and not enough on discovering if there was "something around the edges of those conditions that is really the most important element of therapy" (p. 43). I don't know what Rogers had in mind here, but I for one believe that faith or confidence in an approach seems to me to be the thread common to all therapies. When therapists believe in their theory of orientation, changes occur. In the client-centered/person-centered approach there is more emphasis on belief in the client, but to me belief in the approach is equally important. In addition, I would like to see more outcome articles. Rogers made the famous study with "schizophrenics" in Wisconsin.

7. Do we need more in-depth studies about that "something around the edge" of the "core conditions?" Do you concur with Rogers about that "something around the edge?"

Answer to Questions 7

I would guess what Rogers had in mind in his "around the edge" statement had something to do with trusting the therapist's intuition. In Rogers' article, "A Client-centered/Person-centered Approach to Therapy," in Kutash & Wolf (Eds.) Psychotherapists' Casebook. Jossey-Bass, 1986, 197-208 (reprinted in the Carl Rogers Reader), he describes "one more characteristic…when I am closest to my inner, intuitive self…then whatever I do seems to be full of healing."

I believe very much in the therapist's functioning freely, departing from the "book," as long as there is no systematic direction and there exists a basic trust in the self-directive capacity of the individual or group. Yes, it would be great to have some research on this.

Question 7 a

7 a. Do we also need more outcome studies and what areas would you like to see presented? For instance, I would like to see more on using the person-centered approach with "alcoholics."

Answer to Question 7 a

Yes, I would like to see more outcome studies. I think it would be difficult to use standard diagnostic categories, because person-centered clients are usually not selected this way. I would rely on a phenomenological approach, facilitating clients' responses in their own terms about what brought them to therapy, their experience of the process, and their evaluation of the outcome, and I would use interviews, not questionnaires.

Question 7 b

7 b. Are person-centered therapists spending too much time on articulating the theory and failing to share what we learn from entering the world of clients as if? What should client-centered therapists be writing about? For instance, I believe our interest in the perceptions of clients puts us in a position to tell others what it is like to be schizophrenic, or a child, rather than hearing what "experts" say about the variety of problems people face based on quantitative investigations.

Answer to Question 7 b

I am not comfortable telling other people (including client-centered therapists) what they should be doing or writing about. My answer to 7b indicates that I also favor taking advantage of a qualitative understanding of the client's frame of reference. I would pay attention to individual differences and variance and, as you imply, not be concerned only with measures of central tendency (statistical averages, etc.) or even qualitative generalizations about the population studied.

Question 8

8. What criticisms concerning client-centered/person-centered theory and practice have you encountered?

Answer to Question 8

It is too centered on the individual. Individuals are in relationship, members of families, of cultures and societies. Therefore it doesn't make sense to treat the individual alone.

It is a selfish point of view. People shouldn't be encouraged to do only what feels good or makes them happy, to look out only for themselves.

It is too trusting a point of view. People aren't that good and wise. Clients, students, children sometimes need guidance.

It is superficial. People are influenced by unconscious forces.

It is too intellectual. It ignores the body.

These are criticisms I have encountered. I want to make it clear that I do not agree with them.

Question 9

9. Since you were not the formulator of client-centered therapy, what is your most difficult struggle with articulating and practicing client-centered therapy and theory?

Answer to Question 9

These are good questions. Because I did not formulate the approach, I believe that I have to keep learning from my own experience the effects of different ways of responding to the client. My responses are not always client-centered, because I believe that it is vital to be myself in the relationship. It is therefore difficult to be consistently client-centered on a behavioral level; so occasionally I may make a suggestion, put out my own metaphor, joke, inject something from my own experience, etc.. The result of all this is that I have confirmed for myself that it is most effective to be as consistently client-centered as I can be, within the context of operating freely.

Question 9 a

9 a. What doubts or questions about the theory do you have?

Answer to 9 a

I don't think the approach is as effective with as many people as it once was or as I used to believe. Life (during my lifetime) has become increasingly difficult and stressful, in spite of or because of, all of the technological advances that have occurred. The need for economic and personal security, always strong, has intensified, making it more difficult to believe in one's own capacities and contributing to the reliance on experts and on specific (often behavioral) solutions for specific problems, by individuals and organizations. Perhaps the theory underestimates the need for security. Rogers was very secure in himself and had an amazing belief in others. I guess this is a characteristic of greatness, e.g., Martin Luther King, Franklin Delano Roosevelt.

The difficulties do not mean that I have changed my way of trying to help people. There is a greater need than ever for belief in self, and that is the way I want to practice and teach. I am appalled by the way my profession, among others, has embraced expertise.

Question 10

10. What significant contributions did and does client-centered therapy and practice provide to psychotherapy and education?

Answer to Question 10

* A point of view that remains distinctive and more important than ever.
* Making it clear how to "do it," through verbatim interviews and cases, articles, books, audiotapes, videotapes, films.

* The formulation of a set of principles applicable to education and to human relations in general.
* Lots of evidence that it can work.

If this is the end or whenever we reach the end of the interview, I would appreciate seeing the whole thing in one piece.

Finale'

I had a couple more questions. I decided during the Warm Springs workshop that year not to ask them. There was something about your last set of answers that made it seem like it would be anticlimactic to ask anything more.

The last task was to find a format to present the interaction. Should I make it appear like a face to face interview? Should I try to retain the e-mail format which had a lot of Internet distractions? I decided to offer a combination of both. What have I created here? A blending of two formats, the traditional format of a face to face interaction, and the new format of e-mail communication. Neither on their own would be sufficient to capture the essence of the interaction. To prepare the material in the traditional format of a face-to-face interview would make the interaction appear to be something it wasn't. To present the material in its e-mail format would be cumbersome to read. My hope is that the reader could follow the interaction that took place between Nat and myself. I am excited about the questions and extremely excited about the responses.

References

Bozarth, J. (1987). Person-centered workshop. **Person-Centered Review**, 2(3), 311-314.

Bozarth, J. & Brodley, B. (1986). Client-centered psychotherapy: A statement. **Person-Centered Review**, 1(3), 262-271.

Brodley, B. (1994). Observations of Carl Rogers behavior in therapy. **The Person-Centered Journal**, 1(2), 37-47.

Cain, D. (1986). What does it mean to be "person-centered"? **Person-Centered Review**, 1(3), 251-256.

Dana, R. Q. (1985). Pretreatment assertion levels as they relate to treatment outcome in an alcohol abusing sample. **Dissertation Abstracts International**, 46(3-B), 956.

Obitz, F. W. (1975). Alcoholics' perceptions of selected counseling techniques. **British Journal of Addiction**, 70(2), 187-191.

Pfeiffer, W., Feuerlein, W., & Brenk-Schulte, E. (1991). The motivation of alcohol dependents to undergo treatment. **Drug & Alcohol Dependence**, 29(1), 87-95.

Raskin, N. (1996). Person-centered psychotherapy: Twenty historical steps. In W. Dryden (Ed.), **Developments in psychotherapy: Historical perspectives**. London: Sage.

Rogers, C. R. (1942). **Counseling and psychotherapy**. Boston: Houghton Mifflin.

Rogers, C. R. (1951). **Client-centered therapy**. Boston: Houghton Mifflin.

Rogers, C. R. (1957). The necessary and sufficient conditions of therapeutic change. **Journal of Consulting Psychology**, 21, 95-103.

Rogers, C. R. (1959). A theory of therapy, personality, and interpersonal relationships, as developed in the client-centered framework. In S. Koch (Ed.), **Psychology: A study of a science**: Vol. 3: **Formulations of the person and the social context** (pp. 184-256). New York: McGraw-Hill.

Rogers, C. R. (1986). A client-centered/person-centered approach to therapy. In I. Kutash, & A. Wolf (Eds.), **Psychotherapists' casebook** (pp. 197-208). San Francisco: Jossey-Bass.

Forty Years of Dialogue with the Rogerian Hypothesis

Jerold D. Bozarth

This chapter reflects four decades of my thoughts and experience that involve Client-Centered Therapy/Person-Centered Therapy and the Rogerian hypothesis. What I would like to share is not only what I believe but a bit about how I have come to believe that the person-centered approach is revolutionary and founded upon a different paradigm from other therapeutic approaches. Although the focus of this paper is upon therapy, the revolutionary paradigm is considered to be significant for all interpersonal relationships (Rogers, 1959).

The Different Paradigm

Paradigm refers to a set of beliefs and assumptions that undergird the functional theory. A new paradigm refers to a "new vision of reality; a fundamental change in thoughts, perceptions, and values" (Capra, 1982, p. 16). Rogers' view is different from other therapeutic assumptions including most humanistic views. He assumes a growth hypothesis that is natural and universal which propels individuals towards finding their full potentialities (Bozarth, 1998, pp. 27-34); Bozarth and Brodley, 1991; DeCarvalho; 1991; Rogers, 1961). This is the foundation of the person-centered approach. Moreover, his theory contends that this growth can be promoted by the client perceiving certain conditions that are experienced by the therapist towards the client. I will say this in a different way later, but the implicit practicality for therapy is that the client must be free to follow her own way, in her own direction and at her own pace. It is the client/therapist relationship and the resources of the client that are most important for success.

Some Beliefs

Here are several of my beliefs about Person-Centered Therapy:

1. The therapist must BE a certain way, congruent, in the momentary relationship to the client while experiencing unconditional positive regard towards and empathic understanding of the client's frame of reference.

2. The client must minimally perceive the therapist's experience of unconditional positive regard (UPR) towards and empathic understanding (EU) of the client's frame of reference.

3. The fundamental curative or promotional factor is the client's perception of the therapist's experience of unconditional positive regard. It can be no other way in Rogers' theory.

4. There are no goals of the person-centered therapist for the client. The only goal of the therapist is for the therapist to be a certain way.

5. The primary preparation of the person-centered therapist must be the development of her own unconditional positive self-regard.

6. The primary condition is the growth hypothesis; i.e., the actualizing tendency.

7. The necessary and sufficient conditions hypothesized by Rogers are ultimately one condition in unity with the growth hypothesis.

These beliefs will be elaborated upon later.

First Realizations

My first realization of the monumental difference of this theory occurred for me between 1958 and 1963 when I was in my middle and late 20's. I started my first professional employment as a Psychiatric Rehabilitation Counselor in a State Mental Hospital. I joined a pilot project intended to help chronic, long term "mental patients" find ways out of the hospital. My academic background included an undergraduate degree with majors in social studies, sociology, speech and psychology with little study of counseling or psychotherapy. My responsibility was to develop a psychiatric rehabilitation department and to find ways to help the individuals. At the time, I had not learned the party line of many academicians and clinicians that Rogers' approach "would not work" with individuals who were in "psychotic" states of dysfunction. In fact, I had not even heard of the "Rogerian" or "Client-Centered" approach at that time. The professional hospital staff often assured me that nothing would help these "psychotic" and "institutionalized" individuals to function outside of the hospital. As it turned out, many of these individuals improved significantly to the point of reasonable self-sufficiency outside of the hospital. My observations of this improvement were buttressed by the hard evidence of reduced recidivism rates, functional employment, independent living, self evaluations and increased quality of life. I did not know of the work of Carl Rogers until introduced to me by the director of the pilot project who supervised me from another city. Knowing little about what to do, I depended upon the individuals with whom I worked. I listened, cared for and trusted them. My major interest was that of finding what was effective for the individuals with whom I worked. What was the assumption that created a different paradigm? **The self-direction of the client could be trusted**. The clients, who averaged individual hospitalizations of over twenty years, found ways to improve their lot. What was the revolutionary aspect? **The relationship and the resources of the client were the primary treatment factors**. There was seldom focus on depth of self exploration or experiencing or any other particular process. Here are several examples:

Howard had been hospitalized twenty years before I saw him, diagnosed as, Schizophrenic, Paranoid type. He had stabbed several individuals prior to his admittance. He had a grounds pass at the hospital and worked at a paper route in the hospital. He heard about me from other residents and asked his doctor to refer him to me. We talked twice about his thoughts of getting out of the hospital. He decided that this was not the thing for him to do, too threatening! I mostly listened, told him about some of the training and educational possibilities that I could help him with if he did decide to develop out hospital plans. Nearly a year later, he returned to pick up where he left off. He inquired about the possibility of "Barbers School". We talked weekly for several months with him taking the lead. He talked about his daughter, his relationships at the hospital and things most of us might talk about in normal conversations. His consistency with seeking training resulted in him being accepted for funding to attend such a school. There was a wait period before going to school and he decided to seek employment in the community. Although, it was the height of a recession in an industrial community, I supported his wish to seek employment. We talked before and after trips to the city. Most of the staff were quite skeptical about him finding employment when "normal" individuals could not find even part time work. One week later, Howard had three job offers. He accepted one job as a "prep" person shaving individuals before they went to surgery. Later, he went to the school and worked as a barber until his retirement. I always thought that these were interesting jobs for him since he was originally admitted to the hospital for a rampage with a knife that resulted in injuries to a number of people.

Eleanor was referred to me by a ward attendant. She had been diagnosed twenty one years before as, Schizophrenic, Undifferentiated Type. She was on a locked ward in the hospital. The attendant said that she had expressed an interest in getting out of the ward, and he wondered if I could help her in any way. When I arrived, Eleanor was sitting on the floor playing with her feces. I had no idea what to do or say. I introduced myself and told her a little bit about my role in the hospital. She was not responsive except for a wild black toothed smile as she continued to play with her feces. I stayed not knowing what to say or do. Now and then I asked a question or made a statement of some kind. I tried to experience her as best as I could wondering what I could do to be more sure of my contact with her. In desperation, I finally blurted out something like, "Do you think that you might like to go to beauty school?" Maybe I was reminded of her creativity and manual dexterity as she played with her feces. Amazingly, she discarded her activity with the feces and sat in the chair next to me. I told her I would come back next week to check with her again. A short time later, she began to discontinue some of her bizarre behavior. She cleaned herself up over the next months and moved to an open ward. She eventually worked some in the hospital commissary. I do not think that she ever got out of the hospital but the quality of her life increased significantly.

Gerald was a twenty-one year old who was diagnosed as Paranoid when he entered the hospital two years previously. He received permission from his doctor to talk to me about finding a job. He worked on the garbage truck in the hospital but was periodically transferred to a locked ward because of violent behavior towards co-workers. We sat mostly in silence over a half dozen or so sessions. I would say things to him or ask questions every once in awhile. He would answer briefly, "Yes" or "No" when a binary response was possible. I could often "feel" anger exuding from him. I would tell him occasionally that I was sometimes afraid of him. He kept returning. Six months later, I took him to town while he searched for employment. Eventually, he found a job and was discharged from the hospital. Three years later, I received a letter from him which thanked me for helping him and for having faith in him. It was not the end of my information about him though. Over fifteen years later, I was chairing a graduate program in a State University. I was cleaning up old student files that had gathered years before my arrival as I came across Gerald's name. It had to be him because of his previous residence and other factors. He had been in the military service, honorably discharged and had received his graduate degree in a helping profession. It is still difficult for me to believe that after fifteen years, this coincidence occurred.

What did I learn from my experiences with such individuals? **Clients who demonstrated varied but clear improvements did not usually focus** on their internal experiences; **they did not delve into self-exploration, they did not focus on their feelings.** They, in fact, talked about anything and everything or nothing. There was no particular technique or way of responding that helped them. I describe myself as offering individuals a naive trust in their own self determinations, a lack of presumptions in what they should be or do or become, and treating them as equal human beings in their own rights. **The great learning for me was that the clients could be depended upon to find their own ways of growing.** I learned that I could depend upon the individual for the best direction for her life. I learned and assimilated a trust for the remarkable resiliency of human beings. In retrospect, I learned the therapeutic potency of the relationship and of trusting the client's resources for change.

The Quest for a Helping model

I found the model for my approach when I read Rogers' (1957) hypotheses concerning the necessary and sufficient conditions for therapeutic personality change. The model did not require particular ways of responding, but offered a guideline for therapists' relationships with clients. It fit what I had been doing with these chronic, long term, hospitalized individuals. The therapist could do many things, say many things, and behave in multiple ways while holding certain attitudes toward their clients. These attitudes could exist within a context of varied activities. It was a model which provided me with a way to be an instrument for individuals to improve within a context that was more than but included psychotherapy.

As I pursued higher education, I was trained in therapies that included Adlerian, Psychodynamic, Gestalt, Behaviorism, Cognitive Behaviorism and Vocational Counseling and Guidance. My education in person-centered therapy was informal, self-directed and seldom related to any professional training program. I maintained an abiding interest in the "necessary and sufficient conditions" and in the client-centered approach espoused by Rogers (1957; 1959). **I learned during this venture that students sel-dom had the opportunity to experience the potency of going with the client's way and direction.** All of the other models were "interventive" in one way or another. The other models short circuited the opportunity for the extreme trust of the client.

My quest for a model took a slightly different turn as I started to examine Rogers' work from a more academic perspective. In the late 1960's, and 1970's, I was involved with two immense research projects with the late Charles B. Truax and late Kevin Mitchell. These projects (The Arkansas Projects) entailed the examination of the "necessary and sufficient conditions" of highly trained and experienced psychotherapists and, a separate project, of Rehabilitation Counselors in the United States (Mitchell, Bozarth, and Krauft, 1977). My realizations from this research were (1) that there were few therapists or counselors who operated at high levels of these conditions during their sessions. High levels of empathy or unconditional positive regard as measured by the best available instruments seldom existed. The best levels were moderate levels (3 on 5 point scales). (2) that clients' improvement was most often correlated with the therapist being reasonably real individuals within the relationship. Congruence ratings that were lower than the operationally defined minimal functioning levels related to moderate but multiple client improvements. (3) that the meaning of the Rogerian hypotheses were undertaking a subtle change of meaning. Later, examination of other studies (Mitchell, Bozarth, and Krauft, 1977) confirmed that there were seldom high level condition therapists in the study samples. **I was reminded that usually clients will move forward with whatever they find from their therapists if there is a reasonable relationship of "caring", "acceptance" or "unconditionality" perceived.** Overall, the research results suggested that client improvement was moderate while high level therapists' conditions were a rare phenomenon (For summary of client-centered research, see Bozarth, Zimring, & Tausch, in press).

Three Model Direction

Part of my work on the Arkansas research projects involved the development of one of the first training manuals on what has come to be identified as "Human Relations Training" or "Interpersonal Skills Training" models. The works of Carkhuff (1969) and Truax (Truax and Carkhuff, 1967; Truax and Mitchell, 1971) became the forerunner for these models which are now more behaviorized and prominently discussed by Cormier and Cormier (1991) and Egan (1975) as well as others. My discovery while working on the development of the skill models was that this was a distortion of Rogers' concepts. The concepts were operationally defined for the purpose of research. These operational concepts were then used to develop training programs. What eventually got lost and distorted was the trust stance of the therapist in the client. The skill model deflected the meaning of the conditions as attitudes and set up a model which instructed therapists to "relate, get the client to understand, and then get the client to action", a clear violation of the fundamental trust model of Rogers' theory. The locus of control was shifted from the client to the therapist. My conclusion at this juncture was (and still is) that there are three models emanating from Rogers' theory and statements. I identify these models in this way:

The **Interpersonal Skills Model** (or Human Relations Model), which is problem-centered and therapist driven;

The **Integration Model** (or The Necessary and Sufficient Conditions Model) (Also identified as the Conditions Therapy Theory by Barrett-Lennard (1998), which is conditions centered and may be therapist or client driven;

The **Person-Centered Model** (or Client-Centered Model), which is person-centered and client driven.

I concluded that the Interpersonal Skill Model is a distortion of Rogers' theory even though widely identified as representing the theory. The Integration Model was also often viewed as the client/person-centered model and interpreted in ways that misdirected Rogers' message. Rogers' Integration Model is considered as the core of all effective therapy regardless of the type of therapy. As such, he accepts the communication of the conditions through widely disparate means. Attention to the trust of the client is relegated to less discussion as he focused upon the therapist's conditions. However, the conditions cited in the Integration Model are the critical instructions to the client-centered therapist (Bozarth et al., in press; Rogers, 1959).

The Influence of Groups

I became interested in groups during the time of my work in the State Mental Hospital System. My approach to groups seemed to go against most of the group literature as I depended upon clients for the direction and substance of our activities. Later, it seemed natural for me to become involved in Rogers' (1970) direction of the "Basic Encounter Group" and later the Large Community Group Bozarth, 1998, pp. 149-159). From 1974 until now, I have been consistently involved with person-centered groups including activity with The LaJolla Program, Community groups facilitated by Rogers and colleagues, and person-centered workshops in Warm Springs, Georgia . I have coordinated the Warm Springs Person-Centered Workshop from 1987 through 1999. **I learned from these groups to trust individuals and the individuals as a group, to trust myself more, to absorb the happenings, and to say little most of the time. I came to believe that an atmosphere of freedom, a safe place for individuals to struggle, a place for individuals to be accepted as they are were the main ingredients for growth. Empathic understanding and facilitator expertise seem less and less important for personal growth in groups.** If this were true, I pondered the implications for individual therapy and for the theory

Indwelling the Theory

The theory is a different paradigm! The theory is revolutionary! Why? **It is a different paradigm because of the radical trust in the client and in the notion of the growth hypothesis. It is revolutionary because it flies in the face of other treatment assumptions.** Notably, the assumption of most mental health treatment models is, one way or another, the specificity assumption. That is, there is the assumption that there are certain treatments for particular disabilities. There is a focus on the problem of the client. The person-centered assumptions are that the healing is natural in the client and that nature is promoted by the therapist/client relationship and by the discovery of the client's own resources. Client problems will be solved as the client's growth tendency is promoted. Clients find their own ways of dealing with the problems. As I examined the theory over and over, I acquired more clarity on the nature of this revolutionary paradigm. Again, I will share this briefly through my own historical perspective.

A Reconceptualization of the Necessary and Sufficient Conditions

Something continued to intrigue me about Rogers' great hypotheses concerning "The necessary and sufficient conditions". It struck me that the conditions of congruence, unconditional positive regard, and empathic understanding of the client's frame of reference were usually discussed as separate rather than having the high interrelationship communicated by Rogers' statement. Further, there was something a bit incomplete in Rogers' statement of the necessary and sufficient conditions when Rogers' theory of pathology is considered. My (Bozarth, 1998, pp. 43-49) reconceptualization of the necessary and sufficient conditions for therapeutic personality change entails (a) genuineness (or congruency) being viewed as a therapist state of readiness that enables the therapist to better experience the client with empathic understanding of the client's internal frame of reference and to experience unconditional positive regard (UPR) towards the client; (b) Empathic understanding (EU) of the client's frame of reference being viewed as the action state of the therapist in which the client's world is accepted the client is experiencing it at any given moment. This is the most optimal way for the client to perceive the therapist's experience of unconditional positive regard towards her; and (c) Unconditional positive regard is viewed as the primary change agent in which the client's needs for positive regard and positive self regard being met. This results in congruence between the client's organismic experience and self concept as part of the promotion of the actualizing tendency. **The fundamental curative or promotional factor is the client's perception of the therapist's experience of unconditional positive regard. It can be no other way in Rogers' theory!** Individuals become disturbed or incongruent because of the introjection of conditional self values garnered from parents and society. Numerous authors realize this point which is included in writings by Brodley (1993), Lietaer (1984), Mearns (1994), Thorne (1991) and Van Belle (1990) to name several. The relationship of the pathological etiology has not been explicitly considered in relation to the necessary and sufficient conditions. It is the client's perception of the therapist's experience of unconditional positive regard that allows the client to experience unconditional positive self regard; thus becoming whole again and to open their organismic experiences without distortion or conditionality.

Interrelationship of the Conditions

I (Bozarth, 1997) discovered while investigating "Rogerian Empathy" that Rogers' empathic understanding of the person's frame of reference and unconditionality are integrally intertwined even to the point of being one condition. The client must perceive both of these conditions as experienced by the therapist towards the client. This is clear in both of his formal conditions statements of 1957 and 1959. Rogers rarely discussed empathy without making references to "acceptance", "unconditional positive regard" (UPR) or similar terms. Empathy (EU) was seldom discussed as a separate quality by him. In addition, consideration of precise definitions of each of these conditions suggest high integration. That is, the therapist accepts each momentary experience of the client (UPR) and accepts each momentary perception and experience of the individual's world (EU). Likewise, the overlap of congruence with UPR and EU is also present in a way that suggests that they are functionally one condition.

The Integration Statement

It became clearer that Rogers' 1957 statement concerning the necessary and sufficient conditions was not about Client-Centered Therapy (Stubbs & Bozarth, 1996). This is a fact widely ignored by most scholars even though Rogers is very pointed that the conditions are NOT just about Client-Centered Therapy. The conditions in this statement have to do with all kinds of therapies and with interpersonal relations in general. One implication of this fact suggests to me that we need to re-frame some of our previous thinking. For example, I (Bozarth, 1983) concluded in a previous review of research in the United States that there were few studies of Client-Centered Therapy per se. Studies usually entail a "method" of therapy seldom using client-centered therapists. The studies often focused on "skills" of the therapist rather than the attitudes. The realization that Rogers' statement is an integration statement suggests that most of the research has been directed towards the conditions cited by Rogers and not towards the stance of person-centeredness. This proves to be a somewhat complicated research problem. To some extent, it provides a rationale for the discovery that Rogers' hypotheses had not been adequately tested; that the numerous research findings of the 1960's were less convincing than reported (Mitchell, Bozarth, & Krauft, 1977). It also sheds some light on the much maligned Wisconsin study with psychiatric clients (Rogers, Gendlin, Keisler and Truax, 1967). Several of he therapists, in my assessment, were not particularly dedicated to the client-centered model and were influenced by other models. They found that they could not apply a particular response model which several labeled, "Client-Centered Listening". The study, at the fundamental level , was an examination of the extent to which the therapists were able to hold the core attitudes towards the clients. Like most of the studies which followed this project, the core conditions became "skills" rather than the attitudinal conditions of client-centered therapy. My personal experience with long term hospitalized "psychotic" clients creates some questions for me of the extent of trust that was offered to the clients in this project. Whatever the case, the research direction became a more general inquiry of the common factors (Rogers' necessary and sufficient conditions) rather than on client-centered therapy per se. Barrett-Lennard (1998) refers to this phenomenon as "Conditions Therapy Theory", while Stubbs and Bozarth (1996) dubbed Rogers (1957) article as the "Integration Statement".

The Research

Numerous research studies were directed towards the basic attitudinal qualities hypothesized by Rogers in 1957 (See Truax and Mitchell, 1971). Research reviews suggested that these studies were not as strong as initially reported (e.g., Bergin and Lambert, 1978; Mitchell et al., 1977). This led to a shift of research focus and to an unsubstantiated conclusion that the conditions hypothesized by Rogers were necessary but NOT sufficient. A later qualitative analysis (Stubbs & Bozarth, 1994) revealed more clearly that prominent conclusions about the research findings were predicated upon rather murky evidence. This was especially true concerning the statement that Rogers' hypotheses were NOT sufficient. There was not one valid study which supported this assertion. This was also true for the conclusion that there is adequate documentation for the assumption of specific treatments for particular dysfunctions. It turns out that these findings blends with a significant direction of psychotherapy outcome research (Hubble, Duncan, & Scott, 1999). In a recent review of psychotherapy outcome research, I (Bozarth, 1998, pp. 163-173) offered the following summary:

The conclusion is clear: There is not a research foundation for the underlying assumption of specific treatments for specific dysfunctions. The specificity myth is replete. I repeat Stubbs and my previous comment that the direction of the research continues to prove

"'…'significantly insignificant to help' and often obscures what is most significantly helpful" (Stubbs & Bozarth, 1994, p. 117). The most clear research evidence is that effective psychotherapy results from the resources of the client (extra-therapeutic variables) and from the person to person relationship of the therapist and client. The specificity and systematizing of these variables remain somewhat murky although they do include Rogers' hypothesized variables of the attitudinal qualities. The research on relationship reviewed by Sexton and Whiston supports the conclusion "…that there are significant individual differences among and within clients over time and that these individual differences account for the majority of the variance in counseling outcome (Martin, 1990)" (p. 58). The data increasingly points to "the active client" and the individuality of the client as the core of successful therapy. (pp. 172-173).

The clear conclusion from five decades of psychotherapy outcome research is that the variance accounting for success are associated with the therapist/client relationship and the resources of the client (extra-therapeutic variables) (Hubble et al. , 1999). It is estimated that thirty per cent of successful therapy is related to the former, the therapist/client relationship, and that forty per cent of successful therapy is related to the extra-therapeutic variables of the client (the internal and external resources of the client). Technique accounts for only fifteen percent of the success variance, and another fifteen percent is accounted for by placebo effect. The outcome research was cast in the form of a therapeutic model by Duncan and Moynihan (1994) in a way which, seemingly unrealized by them, is a near complete parallel with the person-centered model.

The Growth Hypothesis: Extrapolation

The results of the outcome research on psychotherapy persuaded me to re-examine the fundamental notion of the growth hypothesis (Bozarth, 1998, pp. 35-42). The suggestion that seventy per cent of the variance of success is related to the therapist/client relationship and to the resources of the client suggests to me that the cornerstone of successful therapy has more to do with clients than with therapists. Thus, I decided to look again at the foundation block of the Person-Centered Approach in the search for clarity. Clearly, Rogers' foundation block is the actualizing tendency of the individual. Rogers (1980) also discussed a more general assumption which he identified as the "Formative Tendency". Van Belle (1990) offers a succinct summary of these assumptions:

For Rogers everything that exists, including human beings, is taken up into this total evolutionary process of becoming. This growth process has its own ends in view and its own organizational principle within itself. It is a syntropic force, it has morphological properties. It forms and reforms itself dynamically (Rogers, 1980). Individuals, as microcosms of this total process, each uniquely have the capacity to form themselves or to actualize their potentials but they have this capacity only insofar as they are open to themselves, thus only insofar as they function as the "organisms" or growth principles that they are (Van Belle, 1985). Here we have the one and only condition that Rogers posits for growth to occur. (p. 49-50)

My view is that the research findings can be explained by this hypothesis. It became more apparent to me that this assumption is also one that helps with understanding some of Rogers' comments later in his life. Rogers refers to times when his therapy relationship "...transcends itself and becomes a part of something larger..." (Rogers, 1980, p. 129).

As Rogers (1980) stated in a personal paper first written in 1974:

...we are wiser than our intellects...that our organisms as a whole have a wisdom and purposiveness which goes well beyond our conscious thought...I think men and women, individually and collectively are inwardly and organismically rejecting the view of one single culture-approved reality. I believe they are moving inevitably toward the acceptance of millions of separate, challenging exciting informative individual perceptions of reality. I regard it as possible that this view— like the sudden and separate discovery of the principles of quantum mechanics by scientists in different countries— may begin to come into effective existence in many parts of the world at once. If so, we would be living in a totally new universe, different from any in history. Is it conceivable that such a change can come about? (pp. 106-107)

Rogers' revolutionary paradigm has implications beyond that of therapy. The extrapolation suggests that the paradigm could take on new and more radical assumptions. It reflects possibilities that go beyond the realms of current thinking (Bozarth, 1998).

A Reframing of the Revolutionary Position

If we look at Rogers' theoretical position in a different frame, the paradigmatic position may become more clear. It can be simply stated: The person-centered therapist must be a certain way in the relationship! This way entails that of experiencing unconditionality (UPR) towards the client. When the client perceives the therapist as being this way, a natural, constructive healing force is promoted in the client.

It took me forty years of clinical work, indwelling of theory, involvement with research projects and varied types of inquiry to absorb what I had learned from the people I worked with in State Mental Hospitals during 1958 to 1963. Here is a recapitulation of my conclusions related to the above statement:

1. **The therapist must BE a certain way, congruent, in the momentary relationship to the client while experiencing unconditional positive regard towards and empathic understanding of the client's frame of reference.** The therapist must be congruent, "a real person" (not holding a

façade). The therapist must EXPERIENCE unconditional positive regard towards the client. Experience refers to, in this case, the therapist's active and personal living through of unconditionality towards the client. The word "experiences" is important in that it is more indicative of the nature of the conditions being part of the character of the therapist in the relationship. The attention is on the therapist's experience towards the client rather than on communication to the client. Likewise, the therapist must experience empathic understanding of the client's frame of reference. The therapist must to some extent experience what the individual's life is like for the individual "as if' the therapist were that individual. These are great demands for the person-centered therapist that call more for therapist's development, especially of unconditional positive self regard, rather than for skills, techniques and ways to do therapy. Indeed, Rogers(1959) theoretical position is that the therapist's unconditional self-regard begets the therapist's congruence and unconditional positive regard towards the client. Further that these conditions beget the empathic frame of reference of the therapist (See Bozarth, 1998, p. 88; Rogers, 1959, cited in Kirschenbaum & Henderson, 1989, p. 253).

2. **The client must minimally perceive the two conditions of the therapist's experience of UPR towards and of EU of the client.** When the therapist experiences these two conditions, I assume that they are communicated in the interactions between the two individuals. (It should be noted that in his 1959 theory statement, Rogers does not indicate that the therapist must communicate these attitudes as stated in the 1957 statement).

3. **The fundamental curative or promotional factor is the client's perception of the therapist's experience of unconditional positive regard. It can be no other way in Rogers' theory.** The reason individuals have difficulty is because of the introjection of conditional self regard from significant others and society. The corrective factor is the development of unconditional self regard through being received with unconditional positive regard by the therapist.

4.There are no goals of the person-centered therapist for the client. The only goal of the therapist is to be a certain way. There is not a goal of experiencing, or of depth of self-exploration or of self-actualization. There is no particular process or behaviors or direction that any particular person is expected to follow. Others have assumed from Rogers' writings that there are certain goals such as experiencing or self-actualization. This appears to come from Rogers' speculations that certain processes and behaviors are apt to occur with the client if the therapist's experience of the conditions are perceived. The error of this misunderstanding is that Rogers' speculations are interpreted as instructions rather than predictions that are apt to occur. The intent then becomes pursue these predictions as goals. This was clear to me in my early relationships with chronic, long term "psychotic" clients who mostly talked about the realities or fantasies of their lives rather than about their problems. This becomes clear theoretically if we think of the foundation of the theory; that is, that there is a natural, constructive process within each individual. This natural process is promoted when the individual perceives the experiencing of unconditional positive regard towards her. Rogers was actually clear about this in several of specific statements. His goal was to be a certain way himself. He then trusted that the client's growth would be accelerated.

5. The primary preparation of person-centered therapist must be the development of unconditional positive self-regard. This becomes clearer in Rogers' (1959) theoretical statement concerning the family. This statement is a shorter version of his theory of therapy. He states:

The theoretical implications would include these:

1. The greater the degree of unconditional positive regard which the parent experiences toward the child:
a. The fewer the conditions of worth in the child.
b. The more the child will be able to live in terms of a continuing organismic valuing process.
c. The higher the level of psychological adjustment of the child.

2. The parent experiences such unconditional positive regard only to the extent that he experiences unconditional self-regard.

3. To the extent that he experiences unconditional self-regard, the parent will be congruent in the relationship.
a. This implies genuineness or congruence in the expression of his own feelings (positive or negative).

4. To the extent that these conditions exist, the parent will realistically and empathically understand the child's internal frame of reference and experience an unconditional positive regard for him.

5. To the extent that conditions 1 through 4 exist, the theory of the process and outcomes of therapy and the theory of the process and outcomes of an improving relationship apply. (Rogers, 1959, cited in Kirschenbaum & Henderson, 1989, p. 253)

This statement permits us to better understand the importance that Rogers accords to PR in his theory. It IS the parent's (or therapist's) experience of unconditional positive regard towards the child (or client) that (1) creates fewer conditions of worth, (2) promotes the organismic valuing process, and (3) promotes psychological adjustment in the child. Moreover, the parent (therapist) must have unconditional self-regard to be congruent in the relationship and, hence, to be able to experience unconditional positive regard and empathic understanding of the child's frame of reference. This statement succinctly describes the condition of UPR as the curative attitude not only for the client but also for holding oneself congruent as the therapist. It is dependent upon the therapist (substituting for the term, parent) having unconditional positive self regard. It is the bottom line of the role of client-centered therapists; that is, to take one's own unconditional self-regard into sessions with total focus on their clients' with no other intention.

Rogers' revolutionary paradigm has numerous implications.

Some Implications

A couple of the implications of the person-centered paradigm are noted in the following discussion.

Ethics

The fundamental assumption of the person-centered approach is also the basic ethical premise for person-centered practitioners. The manifestation of the assumption is that the practitioner is dedicated to the self-authority and self-determination of the client. As such, the principle suggests new interpretations and even different statements concerning ethical standards. Such revision does not suggest fewer ethical restraints, rather it suggests stronger ethical principles and more attention to the nature and substance of professional relationships.

Psychotherapy is the search for and integration of one's own biologically intrinsic and authentic values. Psychotherapy, for Rogers (1961), like Maslow (1962), was a process of recovery of "specieshood" or of "healthy animality," of self-discovery, and of integration leading toward greater authenticity of being and spontaneous expressiveness. This assumption is significantly different from underlying assumptions of most ethical standard statements. Most ethical assumptions in therapy are embedded in psychoanalytic theory. The assumptions are: (1) that therapists must be controlled in their behavior with clients; that is, they can not be trusted; (2) that clients are helpless in their relationships with therapists (and that feelings are often transference towards the therapist); (3) that therapists are more powerful than clients and can easily coerce clients. It is not my purpose here to argue ethical virtues of a different assumptive base. Rather, the implications of the growth assumption for ethical behavior is identified.

The task of the person-centered therapist is to be a certain way and that way involves the maximal experiencing of self-regard of the therapist. It is assumed that this promotes the positive growth of the individual. The difference between the client and therapist is not the therapist's expertise but the therapist's congruence (in the face of client incongruence) in the relationship. It is the therapist's dedication and intent of experiencing the client in certain ways; i.e., with unconditionally and "as if" the therapist were the client. The abiding person-centered ethic is to operate from these attitudinal qualities. This is the way the person-centered therapist strives to "be". Person-centered ethics are predicated on attitudinal qualities of the therapist. When the therapist is this way, the therapist can be trusted to act in accord with the positive growth directions of the client.

Multicultural Diversity

There have been numerous critiques of Rogers' theory in relation to cultural values and, as well, to gender perceptual stances. The position is often taken that Rogers' values were middle class American values and emerged from the U.S. culture which values such traits as independence, individual resourcefulness and materialistic accomplishments. Some parallel is drawn between U. S. Historical events and Rogers' theory which do demonstrate logical influential factors (Barrett-Lennard, 1998). However, I believe that such arguments are misleading in that they (1) ignore Rogers' basic point of theoretical origin which was that of experiencing and observing the people with whom he worked, and (2) that they minimize the essence of the theory as an organismic, natural and universal theory. The theoretical assumption applies to all human species and indeed, to all living organisms (and even beyond: See Rogers, 1980). The qualities of the biological core are intrinsic to the human nature of each individual. Denial and unawareness of the core lead to psychological illness. Evil is a product of social conditioning and reaction to introjected values of conditional love according to Rogers. The more one becomes what one truly is, the less evil one finds within. The more one permits evil feelings to surface the less potent and burdensome they become (DeCarvalho, 1991). Moreover, the more one actualizes, the more one is able to interface with the environment and others even when at odds with strictures of the norm group. The latter point concerning societal adjustment, although not necessarily societal agreement, with particular societal norms for individuals at higher levels in the actualizing process is important in order to understanding part of Rogers' position (1980). When the theory is cast in a way that is considered inappropriate in particular instances, it is usually cast in the format that individuals have learned to "do" Client-Centered Therapy. Elsewhere, (Bozarth, 1998, pp. 97-102; Glauser & Bozarth, in press) it is argued that focusing on how to do person-centered therapy is one of the more inhibiting factors to creating a free environment for the individual. As such, the arguments that CCT can not apply to certain other cultures are predicated upon this way of "doing" therapy. The foundational premise of a universal and natural force is ignored as the basic premise.

Societal Impact

Rogers (1956) discussed the societal implications of his theory in his early books about therapy. It was, however, in the early 1960's that his primary efforts went in this direction. Rogers (1977) wrote a book concerning the meaning of his theory for society. He believed that the most notable influence of his theory on society was related to power and control in relationships. He described the societal influence of his approach in the following way: "Most notably it has altered the thinking about power and control in relationships between persons..." (p. xii). Rogers summarizes the thrust of his approach numerous times in his book on personal power. One of these quotes is an appropriate to communicate the overall idea. He states:

A person-centered approach, when utilized to encourage the growth and development of the psychotic, the troubled, or the normal individual, revolutionizes the customary behaviors of members of the helping professions. It illustrates many things: (1) A sensitive person, trying to be of help, becomes more person-centered, no matter what orientation she starts from, because she finds that approach more effective. (2) When you are focused on the person, diagnostic labels become largely irrelevant. (3) The traditional medical model in psychotherapy is discovered to be largely in opposition to person-centeredness. (4) It is found that those who can create an effective person-centered relationship do not necessarily come from the professionally trained group. (5) The more this person-centered approach is implemented and put into practice, the more it is found to challenge hierarchical models of "treatment" and hierarchical methods of organization. (6) The very effectiveness of this unified person-centered approach constitutes a threat to professionals, administrators, and others, and steps are taken consciously and unconsciously- to destroy it. It is too revolutionary. (p. 28)

Rogers reminds us of the theoretical basis of these key principles. He notes: "From the perspective of politics, power, and control, person-centered therapy is based on a premise which at first seemed risky and uncertain: a view of man as at core a trustworthy organism" (p. 7). Rogers' revolutionary proposition founded upon the growth hypothesis faces us with different ways of thinking, and practicing and being. Person-Centered Therapy and the Person-Centered Approach is a revolutionary paradigm.

Jerold Bozarth is a Professor Emeritus with the University of Georgia, Athens, Georgia

---

This chapter is a revised version of the paper, **Person-Centered Therapy: A Revolutionary Paradigm**, presented at the Seventh International Forum on the Person-Centered Approach, Johannesburg, South Africa.

Parts of this chapter are reproduced from the book:

Bozarth, J. D. (1998). **Person-Centered Therapy: A Revolutionary Paradigm.**

Ross-on-Wye: PCCS Books. Permission for reproduction is granted by PCCS Books.

References

Barrett-Lennard, G. T. (1998). **Carl Rogers' helping system: Journey & substance**. London: Sage.

Bergin, A. E., & Lambert, M. J. (1978). The evaluation of therapeutic outcomes, In S. L. Garfield & A. E. Bergin (Eds), **Handbook of Psychotherapy and Behavioral Change: An Empirical Analysis (2nd edition)** (pp. 139-189). New York: John Wiley and Sons.

Bozarth, J. D., (1983). Current research on client-centered therapy in the USA. In M. Wolf-Rudiger and H. Wolfgang (Eds.). **Research on Psychotherapeutic Approaches: Proceedings of the 1st European Conference on Psychotherapy Research**, Trier, 1981, vol 11 (pp. 105-15). Frankfort: Verlag Peter Lang.

Bozarth, J. D., (1997). Empathy from the framework of Client-Centered Theory and the Rogerian hypothesis. In A. Bohart, & L. Greenburg (Eds.): **Empathy Reconsidered: New directions in psychotherapy** (pp. 81-102), Washington D. C.: American Psychological Association.

Bozarth, J. D. (1998). **The person-centered approach: A revolutionary paradigm**. Ross-On-Wye, England: PCCS Books.

Bozarth, J. D., & Brodley, B. T. (1991). Actualization: A functional concept in client-centered psychotherapy: A statement. **Journal of Social Behavior and Personality**, 6(5), 45-59.

Bozarth, J. D., Zimring, F. M., & Tausch, R. (in press). Research in client-centered therapy: Evolution of a revolution. In D. Cain, & J. Seeman, (Eds.), **Research in Humanistic Psychology** in press. Washington, D. C.: American Psychological Association.

Brodley, B. T., (1993). Some observations of Carl Rogers' behavior in therapy Interviews. **Person-Centered Journal**, 1(1), 37-47.

Carkhuff, R. R. (1969). **Helping and human relations, Vol 1**. New York: Holt, Rinehart and Winston.

Capra, F. (1982). The turning point. New York: Simon and Schuster.

Cormier, W. H., & Cormier (1991). **Interviewing Strategies for Helpers.** Belmont, CA.: Brooks/Cole Publishing Co..

Decarvalho, R. J. (1996). **The growth hypothesis in psychology: The humanistic psychology of Abraham Maslow and Carl Rogers.** San Francisco: The Edwin Mellen Press.

Duncan, B. L., & Moynihan, D. W. (1994). Applying outcome research: Intentional utilization of the clients frame of reference. **Psychotherapy, 31,** 294-301.

Egan, G. (1975). **The skilled helper: A model for systematic helping and interpersonal relating.** Belmont, CA: Wadsworth.

Glauser, A., & Bozarth, J. D. (in press). Person Centered Therapy: Acknowledging the Culture Within . **Journal of Counseling and Development.** Washington, D. C.: American Counseling Association.

Hubble, M. A., Duncan, B. L., & Miller, S. D. (1999). **The heart and soul of change: What works in therapy.** Washington D. C.: American Psychological Association.

Kirschenbaum, H., & Henderson, V. (Eds.) (1989). **The Carl Rogers Reader.** Boston: Houghton Mifflin Company.

Lietaer, G. (1984). Unconditional positive regard: A controversial basic attitude in Client-Centered Therapy. In R. Levant, & J. Shlien (Eds.), **Client-centered therapy and the person-centered approach: New directions in theory, research, and practice** (pp. 41-58). New York: Praeger.

Martin, J. (1990). Individuals in client reactions to counseling and psychotherapy: A challenge for research. **Counseling Psychology Quarterly, 3,** 67-83.

Maslow, A. H. (1970). **Motivation and personality (2nd ed.).** New York: Harper & Row.

Mearns, D. (1994). **Developing person-centered counseling.** Sage: London.

Mitchell, K., Bozarth, J. D., & Krauft, C. C. (1977). A reappraisal of the therapeutic effectiveness of accurate empathy, non-possessive warmth, and genuineness. In A. S. Gurman, & A. M. Razin (Eds). **Effective Psychotherapy: A Handbook of Research**. New York: Pergamon Press.

Patterson, C. H. (1969). Necessary and sufficient conditions for psychotherapy. **The Counseling Psychologist**, 1(2) 8-26.

Rogers, C. R. (1956). **Client-centered therapy (Third edition)**. Boston: Houghton-Mifflin.

Rogers, C. R. (1957). The necessary and sufficient conditions of therapeutic personality change **Journal of Consulting Psychology, 21**, 95-103.

Rogers, C. R. (1959). A theory of therapy, personality, and interpersonal relationships as developed in the client-centered framework. In S. Koch (Ed.), **Psychology: A study of science: Vol. 3 Formulation of the person and the social context** (pp. 184-256). New York: McGraw Hill.

Rogers, C. R. (1961). A therapist's view of the good life: the fully functioning person. In C. R. Rogers (Ed.), **Becoming a person** (pp. 183-196). Boston: Houghton Mifflin.

Rogers, C. R. (1970). **Carl Rogers on encounter groups**. New York: Harper & Row.

Rogers, C. R. (1977). **Carl Rogers on personal power: Inner strength and its revolutionary impact**. New York: Delacorte.

Rogers, C. R. (1980). **A way of being**. Boston: MA.: Houghton Mifflin.

Rogers, C. R., Gendlin, G. T., Keisler, D. V., & Truax, C. B. (1967). **The Therapeutic Relationship and Its impact: A Study of Psychotherapy With Schizophrenics**. Madison: University of Wisconsin Press.

Sexton, T. L., & Whiston, S. C. (1994). The status of the counseling relationship: An empirical review, theoretical implications, and research directions. **The Counseling Psychologist**, 22(1), 6-78.

Stubbs, J. P., & Bozarth, J. D. (1994). The dodo bird revisited: A qualitative study of psychotherapy efficacy research. **Journal of Applied and Preventive Psychology**, 3(2), 109-120.

Stubbs, J. P., & Bozarth, J. D. (1996). The integrative statement of Carl Rogers. In R. Hutterer, G. Pawlowsky, P. F. Schmid, & R. Stipsits (Eds.), **Client-centered and experiential psychotherapy: A paradigm in motion** (pp. 25-33). Peter Lang: New York.

Thorne, B. (1991). **Person-centered counselling: Therapeutic & spiritual dimensions**. London: Whurr.

Truax, C. B., & Carkhuff, R. R. (1967). **Toward effective counseling and psychotherapy: Training and practice**. Chicago: Aldine.

Truax, C. B., & Mitchell, K. M. (1971). Research on certain interpersonal skills in relation to process and outcome. In A, E, Bergin & S. L. Garfield (Eds.), **Handbook of psychotherapy and behavior change**. New York: Wiley.

Van Belle, H. A. (1980). **Basic intent and therapeutic approach of Carl R. Rogers**. Toronto: Wedge Publishing .

Van Belle, H. A. (1985). Humanistic psychology. In D. G. Benner (Ed.), **Baker Encyclopedia of Psychology**. Grands Rapids, MI: Baker Book House.

Van Belle, H. A. (1990). Rogers' later move toward mysticism: Implications for client-centered therapy. In G. Lietaer, J. Rombauts, & R. Van Balen (Eds.), **Client-centered and experiential psychotherapy in the nineties** (pp. 47-57). Leuven: Leuven University Press.

Person-Centered and Humanistic
Theoretical Positions

Ontological Awareness:
An Existential/Cosmological
Epistemology

Bryan Farha

It is common for existential theorists and practitioners to believe that confronting existential issues such as death, freedom, suffering, and meaning is critical in becoming a fully-functioning person (e.g., Bugental, 1965; Yalom, 1980). Ontological Awareness (OA) theory is viewed from an existential/phenomenological perspective: existential in that man's continuous search for meaning and understanding is at the very essence of his/her actions; phenomenological in that it addresses the uniqueness of the individual's subjective perceptions of the world. It is also phenomenological by virtue of its attempt to understand, rather than explain, behavior. Ontology (the nature of being) is inherently subsumed within existentialism (the nature of existence) because man cannot "be" without existing. The awareness of "being" and the subjective meaning attributed to existence, then, is the literal translation of ontological awareness.

Due to the boundariless and multidimensional nature of the human mind, OA theory sees little value in speaking of behavior in absolute and precise terminology—no individual person nor academic discipline should profess to having a complete and unified explanation of human behavior, for total personality understanding is not, and cannot ever be, a solvable puzzle. Personality does not fall within the parameters of solution, for its explanation would then become mechanistic/scientific, or unidimensional. Often referred to as the father of phenomenology, Edmund Husserl (1965) shares his perspective of the concept, which helps clarify OA theory's position: "...A phenomenon, then, is no "substantial" unity; it has no "real properties," it knows no real parts, no real changes, and no causality" (p. 566). The sometimes vague and intangible nature of phenomenology makes it difficult, if not impossible, to view human behavior from a purely scientific perspective. This is frustrating for scientists who seek concrete "knowledge" where only partial understanding, at best, is possible.

Despite its desperate and undying efforts, psychology cannot be a true, pure science because of its inability to produce reliable precision in research findings that the disciplines of mathematics, chemistry, and physics can claim, for example. It can and should, however, be studied using the scientific method, in order to provide research psychology with the most valid and reliable findings possible. Psychology, unlike mathematics (where the computation of any operation always yields the same, precise and exact result), chemistry (where the reactions of any merging elements are predictable and reliable to near perfection), and classical physics (where laws of matter, energy, motion, gravity and force, hold true throughout the universe), simply cannot explain behavior accurately, 100% of the time, and therefore, cannot be a "pure" science. Carl Sagan (1980) supports this notion, "We do not understand human behavior well enough to be sure of the mechanisms underlying these relationships..." (p. 331). Therefore, OA theory sees efforts to explain human behavior in systematic and mechanistic terms as futile. The "mind" is not an anatomical/physiological structure with clearly identifiable parts. Therefore, the complicated apparatus of the Freudian model is rejected.

Ontological Awareness theory holds that no single theory of personality should claim to possess truth, the ultimate state of knowledge. In order for a theory to be legitimate it must be presented with enough subjective and interpretive latitude (theory modification) to allow for the changing nature of existence, and to provide enough flexibility to allow each individual an opportunity to incorporate a significant degree of his/her personal beliefs into the theory under study. Otherwise, the theory is professing truth, which mortal man is incapable of knowing. Ontological Awareness is not a theory concerned with being adopted as a comprehensive doctrine of human behavior, but rather is intended to be used as a platform to assist the personologist or reader to discover and construct his/her own provisional theory.

Realizing that the human personality is too multifaceted to understand in terms of a finite set of fixed principles, OA theory holds that personality development evolves via an integration of primarily three influencing factors: (1) biological, (2) social/environmental, and (3) psychological (housing infinite theory-modification capabilities). This theory focuses primarily on factors that the individual can have a significant influence on regarding personal change.

Ontological Awareness theory recognizes that each human being biologically inherits a genetic code inscribed on the chromosomes of the DNA molecule which contain the blueprints for many of our traits and characteristics. Since each living cell contains the same DNA, the biological influence on personality is then, to a large degree, fixed. Without laboratory intervention, the genetic make-up cannot be changed, and therefore, biological aspects of personality development will not be emphasized in this discussion. But we must be cognizant of the highly influential role that biological factors play in personality development, including the primary instinct of survival. The role of the survival instinct is assumed to be paramount in OA theory.

Similar to biological factors, albeit after birth, we inherit a social and environmental package. There also can be no disputing the impact our environmental inheritance plays in influencing our behavior. It is different than biology in that, to a certain degree, we can alter aspects of the environment. But even so, it is unrealistic to assume that a single individual is likely to significantly change or control the environment, and, therefore, social/environmental aspects of personality development will not be emphasized in this discussion.

An obvious and highly visible influence on personality, the psychological realm is the only factor that can be internally controlled because of freedom of choice—and therefore, will be the principle framework in which OA theory is grounded.

Focus on Present and Future

Ontological Awareness theory recognizes the potential impact of the past and early childhood experiences, but emphasis is placed primarily on the here and now, and to a degree, the future, because being and existence necessarily imply present experience. Focus on the past is seen as limiting, restricted existence which is not conducive to optimal mental functioning.

Structural Constructs

View of Human Nature: Ontological Awareness

Ontological Awareness theory holds that part of the uniqueness of being a member of the human species is that, through advanced cognitive abilities and processes, we are largely philosophical beings. Sometimes masking the awareness of our uniqueness as philosophical creatures are animal-like survival instincts, an integral component of humankind, and an inherent aspect of all living things. But we are a philosophical species aware of being-in-the-world. Ontology, or the nature of "being," and the personal awareness of existence, are at the very essence of our physical and mental presence. Therefore, the central principle in OA theory is that of Ontological Awareness—and man's nature, then, is to increase ontological/existential awareness. Ontological Awareness theory sees efforts to describe man's inherent nature in terms of basically "good" or "bad" as unnecessary, primitive, and a futile use of energy. To profess to be able to solve that puzzle would require a divine understanding that mortal people are incapable of knowing. The frequently heard poker analogy is most appropriate: "We are all dealt a uniquely different hand—it is up to us to determine how we choose to play it." Personalities range in diversity to such a large degree that efforts to determine basic "goodness" will be met with futility. Some of the most basic, fundamental, and important ontological questions or dilemmas that perplex man, at either the conscious or unconscious level, are: What is the purpose of my existence in the world? What is the purpose of the world itself? What force, if any, is responsible for the existence of man, the world, and the universe? Ontological Awareness is further defined as the innate curiosity regarding the nature of man's existence and the personal pursuit of increasing this awareness by seeking answers to ontological questions. The curiosity and thirst for ontological awareness goes beyond the nature of human existence, however. There is also a much broader existential dilemma posed to every individual—that of contemplating why the earth exists at all, and the ensuing questions regarding the purpose of other planets, stars, galaxies, and, ultimately, the entire universe. One only needs to glance but a single time at the sky on a clear night to be ontologically mesmerized at the awesomeness of the cosmos. The celestial universe is an enigma, and this kind of existential curiosity can lead to a lifelong search for meaning, be it conscious or unconscious.

Freedom to Choose, Change Potential

As dialectically reasoning organisms, OA theory holds that every individual has the freedom to choose, often from an infinite realm of possibilities. Recognizing that we are somewhat limited by socio-cultural and legal restrictions—and can incur physical ones—all humans, nevertheless, have an infinite spectrum of "mental" choices. The mental aspects of freedom are seen as paramount to physical ones. Therefore, ultimate freedom is unconditional. Even the most extreme and painful forms of restriction, including those of suffering, sensory deprivation, confinement, even physical torture, offer total mental freedom. Born out of this freedom to choose arise lifestyle alteration capabilities. Existence demands change and is never stationary, but rather is moving, growing, and transcending. Paul Tillich's koan, "Being is becoming" (1952, p. 154) could be interpreted as inferring transcendence, or metamorphosis. The human being, as one of the most adaptable creatures on earth, always holds the potential to change his/her behavior at any developmental juncture, including those of infancy and childhood—the most impressionable of life stages—thereby rejecting the deterministic constructs of Freud. Moreover, in a world that is constantly changing by nature, the human species must alter itself and adapt in order to provide a foundation for healthy survival.

Death, Nonbeing, and Suffering

Resulting from our personal awareness of existence, life, and being-in-the-world, is its dialectical opposite: awareness of death and non-being. This awareness of death's inevitability may very well be exclusive to humans. Another inescapable awareness is the reality that, at some level, all people will experience a degree of emotional or physical pain and suffering. No person is exempt from some form of interpersonal or intrapersonal struggle, be it emotional or physical—although many people choose to mask these troubles, possibly to avoid showing weakness and vulnerability, thereby creating the illusion of happiness. Ontological Awareness theory maintains value aspects, however, in these experiences in that human pain and suffering (1) allow us to decide how to better live our lives more constructively when we witness others suffering, (2) can lend previously undiscovered meaning to our own lives when we suffer, and (3) can provide an impetus for spiritual birth and discovery—defined to the reader's liking. Gordon Allport (1984) not only sees value in suffering, but also considers it as the central theme of existentialism. "To live is to suffer, to survive is to find meaning in the suffering. If there is a purpose in life at all, there must be a purpose in suffering and in dying" (p. 9).

As much as the human species has been conditioned to believe nothing positive can come from death/dying, OA theory proposes that there are aspects of death that will actually produce a healthy type of envy, normally at the unconscious level, in certain individuals. Some who have a thirst for ontological understanding will feel as though the dying person, for example, will have the opportunity to sooner discover answers to the ontologically puzzling questions that have been plaguing humankind since they were capable of higher-level thinking. The dead/dying person may possibly have the opportunity to get answers to the deepest philosophical dilemmas regarding the purpose of man's existence that the living person cannot know. This can, to a certain degree, produce jealousy and envy. Ontological Awareness theory holds that dead people are closer to knowing man's ultimate fate than the living. Maybe the best advice to be derived comes from Plato, who reminds us to practice dying. What did he mean?

Planetary Preservation, Responsibility, and the Collective Human Personality

Adaptable and resilient though we humans are, planet earth is not as fortunate. Owners of the most advanced intellectual capabilities known in the universe, as a species we collectively share the responsibility for planetary preservation. OA theory considers this is the inherent obligation each person holds—as a privileged inhabitant of this fragile world, to maintain and protect the only celestial body in the universe known to harbor life. Investigations of other worlds clearly send us a message of the potentially devastating results of planetary neglect. Global warming on Venus, due to a runaway greenhouse effect, has escalated surface temperatures to a searing 900 F—hot enough to melt lead—and atmospheric pressure to 90 times greater than earth's. Planet-wide dust storms on Mars, which prevent sunlight from entering the atmosphere, mimic the effects of nuclear winter, which would threaten survival of the human species. Nothing short of world peace and the preservation of earth should be the goal and obligation of each individual, and of the entire population as a whole. The collective personality, then, is the sum total of all individual personalities. In OA theory, the physical condition of the planet is seen as the most accurate measure of the collective human personality of all people.

Although with problems such as global warming, water and air pollution, ozone depletion, acid rain, threats to the food chain, and nuclear destruction, our collective personality profile is unfortunately, and obviously, disappointing. At the same time that the planting of trees could be undertaken to absorb the trapped carbon dioxide poisons that are causing a greenhouse effect of global warming, instead we are destroying approximately one acre of forest every second, or 86,400 acres daily.

Earth can be viewed as a living, breathing organism and its inhabitants then, become the collective "self" of the planet. Analogously, applying what we already know about individual personality interpretation, it would seem that the collective personality of the planet would include a destructive component such as a lack of self-respect with severely masochistic tendencies to self-inflict pain—abusive elements would dominate this alarming profile possibility. Would this condition in a human not warrant hospitalization and a suicide watch? What does this reveal about the individual personalities of humans?

Motivational Constructs

Thirst for Ontological Understanding

It is natural for human beings to pursue curiosity—and no person is void from wondering what the meaning of his/her existence is. In fact, ultimately, few would argue that it is the most perplexing question known to man. In OA theory, then, this thirst for meaning and understanding is seen as the central principle of motivation in human behavior. The pursuit to attain ontological understanding constitutes a teleological, or goal-directed perspective.

Microcosmic Blindness

Defined as an avoidance mechanism adapted for the purpose of impeding and denying the search for ontological understanding, microcosmic blindness is characterized by becoming overly driven or pre-occupied with one's immediate world/environment. Many people are "doers" who seem to thrive on being constantly occupied with activities such as work, school, relationships, etc., who, in actuality, are avoiding ontological thinking—possibly as a safeguard against the sometimes unpleasant nature of existential issues. Recalling Tillich's koan, "Being is becoming," Carl Whitaker (1976) suggests that the interpretive inversion, "We keep doing to avoid being," must logically merit validity (p. 154). In other words, we keep ourselves so busy and occupied that we prevent ourselves from becoming and actualizing our ontological potential.

Anxiety

Anxiety can be better understood as being produced by ontological uncertainty, or the likelihood that mortal man will never attain satisfactory resolution to existential questions regarding the purpose of man, the world, and the universe—no matter how much time, effort, and money, are spent in this pursuit. We simply will probably never experience complete ontological satisfaction, in our physical lives anyway, because the questions are basically unanswerable—and possibly by grand design. The answers have eluded man to date, and will probably continue to escape us.

As with anyone who fails to achieve a goal, frustration and anxiety can result. Ontological Awareness theory holds that the single, most anxiety-provoking reality in every person is the inevitability of death and dying. Denial, however, can camouflage the outward expression of this anxiety/fear, or it can manifest itself in other emotional capacities, such as anger and depression. These anxieties, be them death-related or not, can provide the impetus for a myriad of undesirable behaviors, regardless of whether or not they are a part of our consciousness. Ontological Awareness theory contends that death anxiety is, to a large extent, magnified by societal and cultural conditioning. Even to some people who claim to be spiritual, death is often viewed as tragic, rather than as an opportunity to celebrate a developmental transcendence.

Illusion of Happiness

The camouflage/denial element in anxiety is very apparent in what OA theory calls the illusion of happiness. There are countless numbers of people who are either fooled by thinking they are living up to their personal expectations and values, or insist on convincing others of their declared happiness when, in fact, this in not the case. Many strive diligently to become financially well-off in belief that it will translate into happiness, then painfully discovering that only internal processes can accomplish this end.

Another illusion of happiness is that of contentment vs. satisfaction. Sometimes people think they are satisfied when in fact they are only content, which is seen as a goal-directed, but not goal-fulfilled state. Still another goal directed, but not goal-fulfilled illusion is that of immediate gratification as a substitute for happiness. We can easily be fooled by momentary pleasure, but eventually will find ourselves unquenched. The person who chronically complains that the city or town in which they live fails to provide them with enough happiness, stimulation, and excitement, and therefore he/she repeatedly relocates, is a prime example of someone whose perception of happiness is actually an illusion exchanged for immediate gratification needs. Again recall Whitaker's resolution of Tillich's koan, "We keep doing to avoid being."

Image, Habit Maintenance

One of the most difficult challenges facing man's mental health development is acquiring the courage to abandon aged habits, sometimes possessed for the purpose of maintaining an image or identity learned from as far back as early childhood. For whatever reason, be it to gain popularity with social peers or to gain anonymity from them, undesirable elements of the human personality are sometimes falsely sustained by unauthentic strokes of reinforcement by people who do not possess the courage and honesty necessary to promote mental maturity. This image maintenance concept can help to better understand the stagnant behavior of some people. It is true that some want to change this aspect of their behavior, however they feel pulled by the magnet of habit. Human beings have been socially and culturally raised to believe that "getting into the habit" of certain things, or ways of life are positive. It is possible for this to be the case, however, many times the word "habit" represents a negative component which has detrimental effects on personality. We get ourselves into a ritualistic behavior pattern that makes it difficult to escape from once this pattern has been cemented into our learning processes.

Position on Spirituality

Ontological Awareness theory does not profess to have ontological answers, but in a personality theory that is both teleological (purposive) and existential, there is enough latitude provided for a spiritual component—which the individual reader could incorporate, even as the core construct in his/her personal application of this theory, if so chosen. To help determine this construct's personal relevancy, one must ask the following question: Do I believe our existence is accidental? If the answer to this personal question is yes, then reading the remainder of this section is not necessary. If the answer is no, then one has the latitude to consider spirituality as a primary motivational construct in personality development.

Spirituality is viewed by some as a concern with existential questions (Watson, Hood, & Morris, 1988). Depending on how one resolves ontological issues, the role of spirituality in personality theory is strictly a personal one. Ontological Awareness theory holds that ultimate explanations for and against the existence of a supreme being are largely the same. A typical argument rejecting the existence of a supreme creator: "I challenge you to show me one bit of physical evidence of God. If God exists, I'm waiting to meet him. But I won't believe what I can't see." A typical argument accepting the existence of a supreme creator: "The evidence is everywhere. Just look all around you at the trees, the stars, the animals, life. Where do you think it all came from?" Both examples are justifying their positions with visualization, or lack thereof, however, one claims to see nothing, while the other claims to see everything. These kinds of arguments are very typical in "supreme being" debates.

Many cosmologists speak of the universe's origin in strictly scientific explanations, thereby rejecting the infinite regression or the freedom to keep asking "why" regarding origins, although many pure scientists are reluctant to acknowledge its validity. But after satisfactory scientific explanations of the origins of earth, the solar system, and the galaxy itself, the next logical question to be posed to science then becomes, "Fine, but what created the universe and for what purpose?" This question of infinite regression (spirituality, actually) many scientists criticize and avoid because of its unverifiable nature. So to what degree do we keep asking "why?" Speaking of freedom, why can't we keep asking why?

Time-Perspective Constructs

Aging

With age, people often become more ontologically aware, thus altering our personalities in a more emotionally healthy direction. This normally holds true at any developmental stage, from birth and infancy into adulthood, and continuing through old age. With age comes a broader spectrum of experiences and insights, translating into expanded awareness. No matter how long you have lived, you are likely more aware now than you were each previous year. And, with awareness comes subsequent change. It is no wonder, then, that elderly people are, as a whole, some of the most ontologically aware members of the population—and this is reflected by the seemingly peaceful nature that many of them carry—and many of us notice. Because elderly people have increased their awareness to such a great extent since their early years, perhaps this "aura" of peace is the result of progress in striving to resolve ontological issues, such as the certainty of death and dying.

Time and Space

Probably the most enigmatic and nebulous concepts man must struggle with are those of space and time. Definitions are subjective and never precise. Are space and time forever? Are they transitory? Will earth and life always exist? Thus far, human existence is embryonic—earth scientists would remind us that if every event that has occurred in earth's history could be packed into a single twenty-four hour period, human beings would be merely two seconds old. Dinosaurs inhabited the planet much, much longer than we humans currently have. If the evolutionists are correct, dinosaurs ruled earth for nearly 65 million years, compared to a miniscule few million for man. From this perspective, the human species is actually brand new. What was the earth's purpose before the dinosaurs, and life in general? As is the case with everything else, we are still evolving and changing. Cosmology's role in ontology and existentialism is a natural—how can one fully pursue the study of human "being" without ultimately studying cosmological existence? We must each struggle with the vagueness of time and space and develop a personal interpretation of these concepts.

Individual Differences Constructs

Personality on a Continuum

Ontological Awareness theory rejects the traditional categorization and labeling of personality types and mental disorders. To assume that personality types are clearly distinguishable, identifiable, self-contained, and classifiable is to limit and restrict something as multidimensional as human behavior. A person is not simply either mentally healthy or mentally ill. Personality then, is seen as existing on a continuum with an endless array of junctures between each extreme, ranging from well-adjusted to maladjusted. This creates the opportunity to better understand the infinite number of ways that individuals can differ from one another. Back in the early history of psychiatry, mental health professionals adopted the policy of pigeon-holing mental disorders in a rather de-humanizing fashion—a bad habit that has proven difficult to abandon.

Myth of Race and Color

Because of the scattered nature of the continental regions, climatary and environmental conditions for plant and animal survival differ drastically across the globe. This holds true for humans as well. Scorching sun on the African continent, for example, demands skin pigment adaptation in order to survive, thus altering the outward appearance of regional inhabitants. Adaptation is critical to survival. There are numerous other examples of adaptational demands of environment and climate that will alter physical appearance over thousands of years of human presence, thereby creating the illusion that differences exist in personhood. Plant life also takes on different appearances across the globe. But geologists tell us that during the earth's early history the continents were likely united as one supercontinent, known as Pangaea. Had the continents not eventually drifted apart, all land dwellers would inhabit virtually the same terrain, thereby minimizing physical differences of plants and animals ("minimizing" is used because distance from the equator would certainly account for some differences). If the earth scientists are correct about Pangaea, then OA theory contends that man is originally and ultimately one people.

Ontological Significance

One of the mental processes that contribute to the uniqueness of the individual is the frequency of moments of ontological significance (MOS). This can be defined as those extremely personal, perhaps only fleeting, instances in which we experience a magnified degree of respect and awe of the universe for no apparent reason, and no apparent warning for its time of occurrence. Moments of ontological significance could be described as an "existential mesmerism" of our place in the world and the universe. The duration of this experience may be no more than a brief microsecond, or could last several moments—but we have all experienced this sense of total amazement of our existence and place in the cosmos, in which there is an exaggerated feeling of peace and belonging, brief though it may be. The occurrence of MOS may be infrequent for us because of microcosmic blindness. When it does occur, however, MOS creates a special sense of enlightenment for us and can lend insight into dealing with ontological issues such as human pain and suffering. As MOS increases, so to does a sense of inner-peace and belonging.

Theory of Mental Difficulty

Consistent with the view of seeing little or no value in labeling/categorizing personality, OA theory prefers to use the term "mental difficulty" in place of the customary "mental illness." Mental difficulty can result from denying the pursuit of existential curiosity. Constricting one's natural curiosity about man's existence leaves a significant void in making sense out of life. A most frequent example is the individual's (and society's) unfortunate decision to make the topic of death's inevitability a taboo item of discussion and thought. To deny the exploration of such curiosity is to harness the very essence of being, thus leading to existential confusion.

Denial sometimes results from our unwillingness to pay attention to natural existential curiosity. Again, if "being is becoming" and if "we keep doing to avoid being," then this could suggest that we keep preoccupied with our, fast-paced, hustle-bustle, chaotic, microcosmic worlds to avoid discovering and becoming aware of our authentic selves. Existential confusion and frustration arise as a result of an individual's failure to arrive at a satisfactory understanding of his/her ontological dilemmas.

Misconception of Abnormality

The terms "normal" and "abnormal" are often difficult to discriminate. Take, for example, societal conformity vs. personal authenticity. People who are truly genuine, extremely honest, and authentic with themselves and toward others are in the minority. They simply are not as abundant, or maybe as visible, as are people who are socially conforming. Difficult for many is the notion that social conformists are not nearly as genuine, honest, and authentic as the so-called "abnormal" population. There is an aspect of schizophrenia, for example, which OA theory defines as "A retreat from reality, sometimes resulting from a refusal to deal with the artificiality of people and the world; a refusal to be indoctrinated and pressured into unauthentic societal conformity." So-called "normals" are sometimes bothered by people with schizophrenia because the average person is threatened by such a magnified degree of honesty. Most people with schizophrenia are genuinely communicating their phenomenal view of the world to us, yet we refuse to try and understand them. In fact, many people who are said to be psychotic may actually be closer to the "truth" and more at peace with themselves than the so-called "normal" population.

To a certain degree, though, people with schizophrenia are choosing to withdraw and retreat—possibly because of the myth that self-worth is contingent upon social acceptance or professional achievement. To combat this distortion, Don Dinkmeyer offers these words as a reminder to ourselves, "What others think about me is really none of my business" (personal communication, October, 1984). Dinkmeyer may be telling us that external validation is counterproductive to mental health. People with schizophrenia may be different largely because they refuse to participate in a sometimes socially phony world. And, who are we to judge abnormality anyway? From the perspective that our mere existence is miraculous, and the awesome possibility of a supreme architect of the universe, then why is it so difficult to believe that a person could claim to hear voices from, and communicate with, a creator or God? Yet the psychiatric profession probably would have little reluctance labeling such a person: "abnormal— auditory hallucinations with grandiose delusions."

Ontological Awareness theory does not try to justify mental problems. However, some harsh realities do exist that may help us to better understand some people's decision to deviate from customary living styles. Reality tells us that life can be tough. Survival is not easy. It is becoming harder to maintain a high standard of living. Wars have been fought and global nuclear destruction has threatened us. Marital problems are rising and the world is increasingly becoming a more difficult place to raise children. Crime and drugs are prevalent. Peer and school pressures escalate. The list goes on. How does one mentally cope with these seemingly unconquerable problems? Unfortunately, depression, withdrawal, retreat, choosing not to cope, and suicide are alternatives—maybe not preferred ones, but alternatives nevertheless. Is it not each person's decision, ultimately, to chose how to cope—in fact, whether to cope, with these problems?

Theory of Adjustment

The tradition to speak of abnormality in terms of "cure" fosters unrealistic expectations. Despite sensational claims, panaceas for eliminating maladaptive behavior are basically nonexistent. Total disappearance of symptoms, if even possible, are probably better understood by the concept of spontaneous remission. Ontological Awareness theory, therefore, prefers to speak in terms of "adjustment" and "improvement," rather than "cure." People with maladaptive behavior are not machines in need of complete overhauling, but rather human beings in need of belief and attitude adjustments. Psychology should therefore not seek to eliminate maladaptive behavior, but rather seek to reduce its frequency and intensity.

Authenticity

Unfortunately, we have been conditioned to believe that conforming to societal expectations and demands equates with "normal" behavior. This can only be seen as restricting personality development. If this is "health," then what does this say for independent thinking, autonomy, and self-discovery? The human species must be autonomous and unharnessed in order to reach a realistic potential. Ontological Awareness theory contends that psychotherapeutic efforts should be aimed at developing genuine, authentic aspects in the human condition in order to truly pursue mental health. When authenticity is gained/restored in the individual, then the magnitude of life stressors will naturally diminish, thereby increasing the effectiveness of coping mechanisms. In this sense, OA theory can be seen as preventive.

Authenticity requires risk-taking, however, which necessarily infers discomfort. Maybe this is why Tillich titled one of his books **The Courage To Be** (1952). Similarly, basketball legend Julius Erving challenges us to take risks and be courageous, "Unless you dare to put yourself at center stage you can never be great" (Farha, 1985/1986).

Ontological Effort

Approximations toward optimal mental functioning are seen as any cognitive/emotive efforts to satisfy existential curiosity or increase MOS. One must desire to expand ontological understanding by means of cognition, genuinely seeking answers to ontological questions. This can be expressed in several forms ranging from a child's momentary, fleeting thought such as, "If mom had married someone else, would I still have been born?" to the much more sophisticated, profound, and philosophical cognition "If man only exists on earth, then what is the purpose of the rest of the universe?" or "Where does man fit in the grand scheme of the cosmos?"—questions the most learned scientific minds pursue professionally and devote the great majority of their lives to. But, whether it be a childlike thought or a more profound cognition, they both have in common the pursuit of existential curiosity, the most cerebrally cleansing activity there is—and the ultimate tool for a lasting, genuine, internal peace of mind. Mental health can result from an individual's choice not to be indoctrinated to societal conformity, therefore opting to be an independently functioning individual, to be the master of his/her microcosmic world, and to be self-determining, thereby minimizing the need for external validation. With this sort of "ontological confrontation," many underlying symptoms will dissipate without directly treating so-called "causes."

Dealing vs. Coping

Coping is seen as a way of tolerating a problem—a tool for getting by and being able to live with internal struggle. This mechanism is necessary, but not sufficient, for personal growth. What is missing in the coping process is a plan of action component that addresses underlying, rather than surface issues, which OA theory calls "dealing" with a problem. The decision to insulate walls and double-layer windows to tolerate loud neighbors is an example of coping with a problem. The act of walking over to the neighbor's house in a cooperative effort to discuss and confront the situation, however, is an example of dealing with the problem.

Therapeutic Techniques

Ontological Awareness theory views existentially-oriented psychotherapies as being more suitable for effecting long-term change than other therapies because of the assumption that working toward resolution of ontological issues is equated more closely with treating core or underlying problems, rather than mere symptoms. Treating symptoms is seen as effecting short-term change at best, and, in addition, is seen as an invitation for symptom substitution. Admittedly, then, OA therapy, normally takes longer to effect significant behavioral change—however, once this change authentically manifests itself, it will be of a more lasting, permanent nature.

Within the formal counseling setting, one of the psychotherapeutic goals of OA theory is to assist the client in the exploration of existential curiosity concerning the nature and personal meaning of his/her existence. Outside the therapeutic environment, though, a central goal would be to increase the frequency of MOS (moments of ontological significance). Some therapeutic techniques that may be helpful follow.

"Avoid Avoidance" Dialogue

When OA therapists suspect clients to be avoiding ontological issues they re-direct the client to confront and deal with these issues, or help them avoid avoidance behavior. It is all too common for clients to change the dialogue in the therapy session when ontological issues arise. This is a natural occurrence because of the expected discomfort involved in dealing with ontological issues, but "dealing" is a requirement for lasting change. Therefore, it is the responsibility of the OA therapist to develop and maintain ontological dialogue, where appropriate. Thauberger (1981) viewed this issue with enough importance to develop the Avoidance of Existential Confrontation scale and the Avoidance of the Ontological Confrontation of Death scale (Thauberger, Ruznisky, & Cleland, 1981).

Seclusion Therapy

For those trapped in "we keep doing to avoid being," an effective technique to help remedy this problem is to provide an environment that is conducive to the cogitation and pondering of existential/ontological dilemmas. This can be partially accomplished by blocking off personal time each week to secure an environment where there are minimal possibilities for distraction. A drive in the country or a walk in a secluded area are both ways of benefiting from this technique, but the most highly recommended form of seclusion therapy to effect long-term change is that of "marathon seclusion." When feasible, an environment of near absolute privacy for an entire day is most beneficial to help clients ponder ontological issues. Distractive elements are not made available. No telephones, no music, no television, and no books are permitted. The individual hibernates in a place that promotes relaxation, thinking, and contemplation of ontological issues. Clients having a difficult time arranging such an atmosphere may go to the extent to get a hotel room and just sit all day. It is astonishing how much progress can be made at resolving ontological issues with an opportunity to cleanse the mind. It may be a difficult undertaking, as confinement frustration is likely to occur, but working through boredom with discipline is a critical aspect that will enable the client to think about important ontological issues that have previously been avoided. In fact, this may very well be the single most difficult challenge ever confronted by the client. Seclusion therapy is not designed for all clients. It is, however, especially appropriate for clients trapped in "we keep doing to avoid being."

Role of Dreams

Ontological Awareness theory recognizes the enormous capacity of the unconscious. Despite the plethora of research, there still appears to be no clearly understood purpose for dreaming. Further, who are we to profess to know the depths of the unconscious? Insights into the precise roles of dreams are much too vast and ambiguous for clear understanding and continue to elude researchers. In fact, with the actual purpose of sleep still unclear to researchers, how can we begin to claim an understanding of dream content? Dream material can be important in counseling, however, in that they can provide clues to analyze unsatisfied conscious needs. The client, by far, is the most appropriate person to analyze his/her dream. Sole dream interpretation by the counselor is therefore seen as inaccurate, whereas a cooperative analysis between the counselor and the client can be insightful.

Conclusion

In the conclusion section of an existential paper on personality, it seems appropriate to address global needs of the collective human personality of all mankind. While Ontological Awareness theory does not suggest panaceas for mental "health," it may be useful to discuss the broadest, most global suggestions for the mental health and condition of the world, as well as expected reactions and criticisms of a theory such as this.

Addressing specific world problems is seen as analogous to treating symptoms, rather than causes in psychotherapy, therefore, OA theory sees efforts to deal directly with global concerns as futile. The strategy of specifically addressing problems of drug abuse, crime, environmental concerns, war, etc., is viewed as treating symptoms of much deeper issues. These problems, then, would be more effectively approached from the following perspective: "What psychological issues/stressors are present that are increasing the likelihood of our choosing drugs, violence, etc., as a means of coping with intrapersonal problems?" Global or world problems are nothing more than the sum total of individual problems.

For OA theorists, the use of vague and nebulous concepts, as well as the lack of empirical testability, will not be viewed as shortcomings or evidence of the incompleteness of this theory—rather these criticisms are expected. Psychology must move their thinking modality so as to get away from maintaining that verification and testability are mandatory prerequisites for a theory to be considered "bonafied." In fact, verification does not lend itself to this type of investigation. This posture should be reserved for pure sciences such as chemistry, physics, and mathematics. Psychology must, therefore, transcend its currently accepted methods for measuring scholarly progress in personality theory construction or this arena of the behavioral "sciences" will remain stagnant—primarily because of the discipline's own stubbornness, egocentricity, and delusional thinking. Otherwise, to achieve the goal presently being pursued by behavioral researchers—that of a comprehensive explanation of personality—would require a flawless "grand unified theory," borrowing physics terminology. In fact, there is a parallel between psychology and physics in that the former is attempting to understand the mind—an extremely broad effort that seemingly is infinitely encompassing, while the latter is attempting to understand the universe, maybe the only discipline which is more expansive than psychology. Physicist Steven Hawking, probably closer to unlocking the mysteries of the universe and its origin than any other scientist, makes this comment on the subject, "…but can there really be such a unified theory? Or are we perhaps just chasing a mirage?" (Hawking, 1988, p.165). This statement is possibly profound and may be applicable to psychology. A grand unified theory of personality is not, and cannot ever be possible in the pure scientific sense by the very nature of the human mind and brain. Any and all efforts to achieve a comprehensive explanation of behavior will be met with futility. Square pegs do not fit into round holes—an invitation to learning that much of scientific psychology has, thus far, declined to accept.

This theory, then, will optimistically meet the expected criticism that OA is not comprehensive in scope, that it does not explain human behavior, that it does not lend itself to empirical testing, and that it cannot reliably "predict" behavioral outcomes. But there simply is little, if any, "order" to personality. To the "scientific" purists in psychology, a simple, yet critical message: life is change. To grow we must change with time. Avoid pursuing the unattainable. There are a plethora of questions in need of investigation on human personality in which testability and verification should be given secondary consideration.

A bonafied effort at a grand unified theory of human personality would be too complicated for psychology to attempt alone, if at all. In fact, maybe this theory of personality would be more appropriate if it were mainly under the domain of philosophy rather than psychology. But in the final analysis, all of the behavioral/social sciences combined could not adequately meet the challenge of explaining human behavior accurately. A multidisciplinary effort on the parts of psychology, philosophy, sociology, biology, chemistry, anthropology, religion, and cosmology, to name but a few, would be an interesting endeavor. But even this joint effort, on the grandest scale, would certainly prove frustrating, and ultimately, futile.

Bryan Farha, Ed.D., is an Associate Professor of Counseling Psychology and Director of Graduate Study in Counseling in Oklahoma City University.

References

Allport, G. W. (1984) Preface to Victor Frankl's **Man's search for meaning** (3rd ed.). New York: Simon & Schuster.

Bugental, J. F. T. (1965). **The search for authenticity.** New York: Holt, Rinehart, and Winston.Farha, C.B. (1986). The relationship of race to the locus of control among collegiate and high school football players (Doctoral dissertation, University of Tulsa, 1985). **Dissertation Abstracts International, 46,** 2231A.

Husserl, E. (1965). In J. F. Rychlak (Ed.), **Introduction to personality and psychotherapy,** (p. 566). Boston: Houghton Mifflin.

Sagan, C. (1980). **Cosmos.** New York: Random House.

Thauberger, P. C., Ruznisky, S.A., & Cleland, J. F. (1981). Avoidance of existential-ontological confrontation: A review of research. **Psychological Reports, 49,** 747-764.

Tillich, P. (1952). **The courage to be.** New Haven: Yale University Press.

Watson, P. J., Hood, R. W., & Morris, R. J. (1988). Existential confrontation and religiosity. **Counseling and Values, 33**(1), 47-54.

Whitaker, Carl (1976). In P. Guerin (Ed.), **Family therapy: Theory and practice,** (p. 154). New York: Gardner Press.

Yalom, I. D. (1980). **Existential psychotherapy.** New York: Basic Books.

The Actualizing Tendency Concept in Client-Centered Theory

Barbara Temaner Brodley

The paper explicates Carl Rogers' actualizing tendency concept. A distinction is made between its action at the organismic level and at the level of the conscious person. The paper emphasizes four aspects of the concept. (1) The actualization tendency is the sole motivational construct in client-centered theory. It is the motivation for individual maintenance, growth, development and healing. (2) Although the actualization tendency has constructive directionality, it does not guarantee positive outcomes. Favorable and unfavorable circumstances, both internal and external to the organism, influence the result of actualization processes. (3) Motivation is inherently directed towards emotional healing, constructive change and maintenance of the whole person. Given this organismic constructive motivation, psychotherapy need not attempt to motivate or guide the client. Client-centered therapy, consequently, is facilitative but not directive. (4) The actualizing tendency is a concept in the domain of the natural sciences, not a moral or ethical concept. Rogers' observed that clients choose constructive directions under the circumstances of a client-centered relationship. This is explained as the result of the actualization tendency interacting with pro-social human potentialities. Client-centered therapy is favorable to the realization of human innate pro-social nature.

The Concept

The actualizing tendency is the sole motivational concept in Rogers' theories. It is a concept that applies to all organisms as well as humans. It is a source of energy and a source of direction. It is associated with the life of organisms. Rogers (1980) wrote:

All motivation is the organismic tendency toward fulfillment. There is one central source of energy in the organism. This source is a trustworthy function of the whole system rather than some portion of it: it is most simply conceptualized as a tendency towards fulfillment, toward actualization, involving not only the maintenance but also the enhancement of the organism (p. 123).

The actualization tendency is a meta-motivation in Rogers' theory. All specific motives, needs and drives are expressed through the actualization tendency. Rogers' actualization theory is different, for example, from Maslow's (1970) self-actualization theory. Motivations conceptualized by Maslow as deficiency needs, i.e., the physiological needs, needs for safety, belonging, love and esteem are included in Rogers' actualization tendency concept. As a person functions in the world, specific needs and motivations become experientially and behaviorally salient. Their energy, their form, and their relation to other aspects of the person are shaped by the actualization tendency and by inner and outer circumstances.

Characteristics of the Actualizing Tendency in Rogers' Theory

The actualizing tendency is a motivational and directional principle. Its major characteristics are as follows:

1. The actualizing tendency is individual and universal (Rogers, 1980). The expression of the tendency is always unique to individuals and at the same time it is a motivating tendency in all organisms.

2. The actualizing tendency is holistic (Rogers, 1959). The functioning of the tendency is a highly fluid, changing gestalt. Different aspects of the person assume figure and ground relations depending upon the specific

aims of the person, and depending upon the immediate demands of the environment. The actualizing tendency functions throughout all of a person's systems. It is expressed in a variable, dynamic and fluctuating manner through the subsystems of the whole person while maintaining the person's wholeness and organization.

3. The actualizing tendency is ubiquitous and constant (Rogers, 1963; Rogers & Sanford, 1984). It is the motivation for all activity, at all levels of function within the person, under all circumstances. It is intrinsic to the moment by moment living of the person. The actualizing tendency is intrinsic to the person's moving, responding, maintaining wholeness, feeling, thinking, striving, self-preserving.

All capacities express the actualizing tendency. The actualizing tendency is operative under all circumstances. It functions when circumstances are favorable and when they are unfavorable to the maintenance or enhancement of the individual. It is the life force of the individual organism. If the person is alive, the actualizing tendency is functioning. If the actualizing tendency is functioning, the person is alive. Rogers (1977) commented in this vein:

This is the very nature of the process we call life. This tendency is operative at all times, in all organisms. Indeed it is only the presence or absence of this total directional process that enables us to tell whether a given organism is alive or dead (p. 239).

4. The actualizing tendency is a directional process. It is constructive. Its constructive direction has two aspects. One, there is an overriding organizational directive process. The actualizing tendency is always directed toward maintaining a person's integrity and organization. It involves assimilation and differentiation processes while maintaining the wholeness of the person. Two, the actualization direction is towards realization, fulfillment and perfection of inherent as well as learned capabilities and potentialities of the individual (Rogers, 1963). The actualization process is a selective process in that it is directional and constructive. It tends to maintain and enhance the whole organism/person. Rogers (1977) wrote:

Whether the stimulus arises from within or without, whether the environment is favorable or unfavorable, the behaviors of an organism can be counted on to be in the direction of maintaining, enhancing and reproducing itself (p. 239).

5. The actualizing tendency is tension increasing (Rogers, 1959). The organism/person is not a drive reduction system. The organism is a system that inherently and spontaneously increases tension levels to expand, grow and further realize inherent capabilities. Reduction of tensions is a secondary, organismic corrective reaction. The overriding directional process is one of tension-increase for the sake of expansion and development.. The growthful directionality of the actualizing tendency requires tension-increase.

6. The actualizing tendency is a tendency toward autonomy of the person and away from heteronomy (Rogers, 1963). The person moves inherently toward self-regulation and self-determination, and away from being controlled.

7. The actualizing tendency is vulnerable to environmental circumstances (Rogers, 1980; Rogers & Sanford, 1984). There are environmental circumstances that are optimal for each individual. There are circumstances that are not optimal but are nevertheless adequate. There are also environmental circumstances that are totally inadequate or destructive to individuals. Some optimal and adequate circumstances are species general and some unique to the individual. Circumstances may be physical, social or psychological.

Although the actualization tendency is inherently constructive, the living person's behavior at any moment is also a result of innate characteristics, learned characteristics and external circumstances. The dynamic interaction of the actualizing tendency with the other causes of behavior may or may not result in what would usually be considered constructive outcomes.

Optimal actualization of a person's nature requires many different, highly favorable and ongoing circumstances. Optimal actualization is a rare phenomenon. Most circumstances range from the utterly deprived or destructive to a relatively adequate range. Human lives are lived in complex circumstances. Different potentialities are affected differently by the same circumstances. over In addition, circumstances change over the life span. The circumstances lived by many persons are not appropriate for a full development.

The actualizing tendency, nevertheless, persists and is not less present, or less functional, under unfavorable circumstances. The tendency's expression in the person's characteristics and in the persons functioning may be more or less distorted or stunted depending upon the circumstances. Rogers uses the metaphor of the potato sprout in the dark cellar growing toward a spot of light to describe the actualizing tendency's persistence and its vulnerability. Rogers (1980) wrote:

These sad spindly sprouts would grow 2 or 3 feet in length as they reached toward the distant light of the window. The sprouts were, in their bizarre, futile growth, a sort of desperate expression of the directional tendency....They would never become plants, never mature, never fulfill their real potential. But under the most adverse circumstances, they were striving to become (p. 118).

8. The concept "self-actualization" in Rogers' theory (1959) refers to the actualization tendency manifest in the "self", a subsystem that becomes differentiated within the whole person. The "self" concept is essential to Rogers' (1951; 1959) theories of the development of normal personality and development of psychological disturbances. He theorizes that under unfavorable conditions, the actualization of the self sub-system may become discrepant from and in conflict with organismic experiencing. Such conflict diminishes and alters the person's wholeness and integration. Consequently, the person experiences emotional disturbance. Alternatively, under favorable developmental circumstances, persons remain open to experience. They develop a self-concept that is harmonious with organismic experiencing. This psychological situation fosters the person's wholeness, integration and feeling of well-being.

9. The concept of consciousness—specifically the capacity for self-awareness—is a salient human channel of the actualizing tendency (Rogers, 1980). Self-awareness gives the person a great range of choices for self-regulation. It permits the development of potentials that may not exist in other organisms.

10. Human beings have a social nature. Consequently, a basic direction of the actualizing tendency in humans is toward constructive social behavior (Rogers, 1982). Human social nature is as fundamental as self-preservation and sexuality, and like these other fundamental characteristics there are individual differences in its strength and in the forms of its expression. Also, like these other fundamental characteristics, it can be over-ridden by other aspects of human nature. And it can be distorted or suppressed by certain unfavorable circumstances. Human social nature is complex. It involves a mixture of innate capacities. These include:

(a) Capacity for identification leading to sympathy. A natural ability to identify with other human persons and, consequently, to feel concern for the welfare of other persons.

(b) Capacity for empathy. Ability to imagine, understand or, through interaction, to engage in the experiences of another and to feel interested in them.

© Care-taking, protective impulses. Tendencies to care for and protect other humans, particularly those more vulnerable or weak, especially infants and children.

(d) Affiliative needs. Tendencies to place oneself in proximity to, and interact with, other humans. Tendencies to need and seek companionship. Tendencies to create social units for mutual satisfaction, protection and in order to meet needs for nourishment and shelter.

(e) Tendencies towards social cooperation and collaboration for the sake of common goals. These tendencies necessarily involve capacities for self-restriction and for encroachment (Goldstein, 1940) in relation to others. Goldstein asserts these tendencies as essential to human individuality, remarking, "Individuality never means simply *I am* but always that simultaneously with me there exist other creatures (p. 201).

(f) Capacities for and inclinations towards forming moral rules and struggle to live according to them.

Note that the first seven of the characteristics of the actualizing tendency described above are common to all organisms including humans. Characteristics eight, nine and ten are most developed, perhaps unique, within humans.

Rogers' idea of the actualizing tendency is almost identical to the drive for self-actualization posited by Kurt Goldstein (1939) in his organismic theory. Some elucidation of Goldstein's theory may help to clarify Rogers' concept.

Goldstein's Actualization Concept

Organismic theory emerged as a way of accounting for and integrating the phenomena of normal and pathological phenomena in humans. Goldstein studied brain damaged World War I veterans. He dealt with his data in a distinctive and creative manner that was unlike Freud's methods. And unlike the methods of the reflex psychologists. These theorists generalized directly from pathological or experimental conditions to the normal. Goldstein recognized a principle that could account for both pathology and for normalcy while distinguishing the mechanisms of the two paths. Pathology, in Goldstein, is a serious deviation from the normal manner of function, but one that manifests the same basic motivation and directionality. Goldstein (1939) wrote:

An organism is governed by the tendency to actualize, as much as possible, its individual capacities, its 'nature' in the world. This tendency to actualize 'itself' is the basic drive, the only drive by which the life of the organism is determined. This tendency undergoes in the sick human being a characteristic change. The patient's scope of life is reduced in two ways. 1. He is driven to utilize his preserved capacities in the best possible way, 2. He is drive to maintain a certain state of living, and not to be disturbed in this condition. Therefore sick life is...very bare of productivity, development, and progress and bare of the characteristic particularities of normal organismic and especially human life. Frequently, maintaining the existent state—the self-preservation—is considered the basic law of life. I believe such a concept could arise only because one had assumed, as a starting point, the experiences in abnormal conditions or experimental conditions. The tendency of normal life is toward activity and progress. Sometimes the normal organism also tends primarily to avoid catastrophes, and to maintain a certain state which makes that possible; but this takes place under inadequate conditions and is not at all the usual behavior. (pp. 196-197)

Thus, Goldstein accounts for reduced and distorted behavior of organisms, including humans. It is a result of inadequate conditions or of organic defects, or a combination of those two factors. The basic tendency of the organism, in such circumstances, is nonetheless the organism's tendency to realize its nature as best it can.

Potentialities and Circumstances

Persons always function according to the organismic actualizing tendency principle. They are constantly actualizing their natures as well as their circumstances permit. The more favorable the circumstances are in respect to a person's innate nature, the more favorable the outcomes. Under very favorable circumstances a person is physically and psychologically healthy and many of the person's potentialities are highly realized.

The concept of potentialities is extremely complex. Potentials are capabilities that are not fully developed. Within one individual there are always a multitude of potentialities. Potentials are organized in various ways within an individual, depending upon circumstances. Development and expression of some capabilities, such as language, tend to be desirable for the further realization of the whole person under almost all circumstances.

Other capabilities, such as the ability to behave without feeling certain emotional reactions, as in performing surgery, are only desirable under specific circumstances. The realization of certain potentials preclude the highest development of others within the temporal limits of a life. Some potentials are capacities for coping with emergencies or other special circumstances. Some potentials are capacities for ongoing living. Other potentials are special talents or gifts.

Realization of potentialities as the result of the actualization tendency involves a complex organization of subsystems within the whole person. Successful realization involves the appropriateness of the context to the capability. It involves the intrinsic relation of the capability to survival or to enhancement of the whole person. Gagging and vomiting are capabilities that are part of the human behavioral repertoire. But these capabilities are usually expressed only under specific unfavorable circumstances. They would jeopardize well-being, even existence, if expressed under normal circumstances. The directionality of the actualizing tendency is manifest in subsystem relationships and the relations of particular characteristics to the whole person. The actualization tendency results in some manner of integration and organization, regardless of circumstances. It may maintain integration and organization by sacrificing certain functions if circumstances require it.

A person's best realization may not be a very good one. There are a number of different categories of unfavorable circumstances that result in poor realization. Unfavorable circumstances include external conditions and internal conditions. External inadequate conditions for the human organism may be immediate or ongoing conditions imposed upon a person, such as physically or emotionally depriving, punishing or traumatic circumstances. Deviations from the normal outcomes of actualization also may result from physical damage, to which humans are susceptible from conception until they die. The result of external inadequate conditions may be a diminished development or impaired integration. Or it may involve socially destructive reactions. The actualization tendency is none the less the motivating force and direction in the person under unfavorable circumstances.

Unfavorable conditions may be internal. Internal conditions leading to restricted development or destructive behavior may involve internalized concepts, feelings and attitudes. Unfavorable internal conditions may have been fostered in a person's early social environment. Rogers accounts for some diminished or distorted results of the actualization process in terms of inadequate, usually internal and learned, psychological circumstances. These learned, internal circumstances are termed "conditions of worth" (Rogers, 1959). Conditions of worth result in distortion and denial of experience. They influence and limit normal constructive outcomes of the actualization tendency

Other internal unfavorable conditions affecting organismic and personal realization involve organic (biogenic) anomalies. These include schizophrenia, manic depressive illness, obsessive compulsive disorder, depressive and anxiety disorders, hyperactive disorders, autism, Tourettes syndrome and some forms of sociopathy as well as many other mental and physical defects and disorders. Biogenic conditions, of course, may be complicated by unfavorable psychosocial factors. Often the person with inherited or organic defects of the nervous system is further injured by ignorant, unsympathetic or outright hostile personal relationships or by destructive cultural policies.

It may seem paradoxical. Nevertheless, the poorly realized person is as much motivated by the actualization tendency as the highly realized person. Actualization is identified, in Goldstein's theory and in Rogers' theory, with the life of the person. It preserves the life and integrity of the person and motivates further self-development, as much as possible, whatever the circumstances.

The Actualization Tendency in the Conscious Person

Human organisms have a characteristic that distinguishes their actualization processes from those of other organisms. This feature makes the actualization theory seem more complicated when applied to humans. As is the case with all organisms, internal and external circumstances influence a person's actualization processes (as discussed above). Circumstances affect the outcomes of actualization motivation.

The actualization tendency is expressed through the human capability for self-awareness and conscious choice. Choices may modify the manner of action and the effects of circumstances on the person. They may produce a different result or outcome of the actualization tendency. For example, a person may know he becomes irritable when he has not had enough sleep. He may choose to take nap. If he cannot do that, he may choose to avoid other people. If he cannot do that, he may inform his companions of his irritable tendency. He informs them to give them perspective that might make his irritability less hurtful. Humans have the potential, through making choices, to correct for at least some of the action of the forces that act within them and upon.

The potential for conscious choice is sometimes referred to as "free will". Free will, however, is not entirely free. It is very likely that a person will not be fully aware of the internal and external circumstances influencing her conscious choices. Persons make conscious choices, for example, without having a fully evolved self-awareness. Decisions that are destructive to the self or to other persons may result from many factors. From an uninformed perspective about oneself or about the situation, from incomplete information, from errors in reasoning, or from unconscious tendencies.

Many internal and external factors, as well as the unforeseeable, often make it impossible for a person to know whether a choice is constructive. In addition, under certain circumstances a person may not want a constructive outcome. Human self-awareness and capacity for choice gives persons great flexibility. It extends human personal and social potentialities. It does not, however, guarantee constructive outcomes any more than does the actualizing tendency itself.

Given the nature of consciousness and the potential for making choices, the actualizing tendency does not operate in a relatively spontaneous organismic fashion in the lives of humans. The wisdom of the organism, expressed in part by the actualizing tendency, may be contradicted or opposed by human conscious choices. Persons may or may not be aware that their choices have been influenced by circumstances that are unfavorable to them.

Client-centered therapy is nondirective and promotes clients' freedom of choice. Clients in this therapy make constructive choices. These constructive free choices are part of Rogers' evidence for the actualizing tendency.

Development of the Actualization Concept

The actualization tendency is the basic concept in Rogers' client-centered theories of psychotherapy, interpersonal relations, personality development, personality disintegration (Rogers, 1959). It is also a basic concept in applications of the person-centered approach (Rogers, 1980). The actualization concept developed from Rogers' experience as a therapist. Rogers was sensitive to evidence of an inherent growth motivation from early in his career as a psychologist and psychotherapist. In an early book Rogers (1942) stated:

Therapy is not a matter of doing something to the individual, or of inducing him to do something about himself. It is instead a matter of freeing him for normal growth and development. (p. 29)

As discussed above, the actualizing tendency does not guarantee an optimal realization of the person. Rogers (1980) wrote: "The actualizing tendency can, of course, be thwarted or warped, but it cannot be destroyed without destroying the organism" (p. 118).

The inherent motivated tendency to grow and develop psychologically may have stunted, distorted or unrealized results. Consequently, persons may be psychologically impaired in many ways. Interpersonal provision of the client-centered therapeutic attitudes facilitates psychological development. It breaks through or unblocks the stoppages and distortions in the psychological expression of the actualizing tendency. Rogers (1980) wrote:

The central hypothesis of this [client-centered] approach [is that] individuals have within themselves vast resources for self-understanding and for altering their self-concepts, basic attitudes, and self-directed behavior; these resources can be tapped if a definable climate of facilitative psychological attitudes can be provided. (p. 115)

These attitudes include respect for the client, trust in the client's inherent capabilities for growth, a nondirective attitude and the therapeutic attitudes—congruence, unconditional positive regard and empathic understanding of the client's internal frame of reference (Rogers, 1957). Clients change therapeutically when a therapist consistently provides the totality of these attitudes at a high level. Research evidence supports the therapeutic efficacy of Rogers' therapeutic attitudes (Cartwright, 1957; Patterson, 1984; Stubbs & Bozarth, 1994).

Rogers was especially attuned to evidence that psychotherapy clients do not benefit, or the gains are soon lost, when they have been guided or directed. Nevertheless, the actualizing tendency concept was a conclusion, not an a-priori position in Rogers' development as a therapist. It emerged out of his therapy experiences. Rogers gradually formed the concept as an axiom in client-centered theory. It functions as a first principle. It cannot be proved or disproved although it is supported by evidence. Rogers (1986a) explained:

In client-centered therapy, the person is free to choose any directions, but actually selects positive and constructive pathways. I can only explain this in terms of a directional tendency inherent in the human organism— a tendency to grow, to develop, to realize its full potential. (p. 127)

Rogers asserts that persons make constructive choices under the circumstances of client-centered therapy. This phenomenon, that is part of Rogers' evidence for the existence of the actualizing tendency, requires explanation.

Constructive Choice in Therapy

Consciousness, particularly self-awareness, permits humans to make conscious choices. As discussed earlier, persons' conscious choices may be constructive or unconstructive. They may result in events that are favorable or events that are unfavorable to the person or to others. The explanation for constructive choices in client-centered therapy involves several factors.

First, all aspects of client-centered therapy are understood in terms of process. Clients' choices in the process of therapy are not evaluated as discrete choices. Choices are processes of choice. They involve sequences of interactions. The sequences involve specific choices, actions stemming from the choices and observations of consequences. These sequences also include feelings about the consequences, and further choices. Clients do not simply make constructive choices. They engage in self-correcting processes or "pathways" (Rogers, 1986a, p. 127).

Secondly, other ongoing therapeutic effects facilitate constructive choices in therapy. Clients' decreased defensiveness, increased openness to experience, greater flexibility towards creating solutions to problems and increased flexibility in behavior (Rogers, 1961). All contribute to the process of constructive choices. Openness and flexibility promote constructive outcomes of actualization process through choice and other processes, in and out of therapy.

Third, the favorable circumstances of client-centered therapy are the relationship climate created by the therapist together with the client. The climate is the result of (a) the therapist providing the conditions of congruence, unconditional positive regard, empathic understanding and the nondirective attitude and (b) the client perceiving safety and freedom in the relationship. All together, these conditions are facilitative and freeing for the client's capabilities for finding solutions to problems and changing unwanted patterns of behavior. Clients' open themselves to alternatives. They change. They abandon their unconstructive patterns of behavior and their unconstructive assumptions and concepts.

Fourth, the pro-social innate nature of humans is a necessary element in the positive and constructive choices made by clients in client-centered therapy. Actualization of the client's innate pro-social potentialities (for sympathy, empathy, care-taking, social affiliation, cooperation and sense of morality or ethics) must be involved in those choices. If humans did not possess a pro-social nature, the freeing effects of client centered therapy would tend to result in self-centered and self-seeking solutions and behaviors. We would observe tendencies towards making selfish choices, at the expense of others. This is not, however, what happens. Instead, clients tend to improve their relationships (Rogers & Dymond, 1954).

Actualization—A Natural Science Concept

Rogers' (1986a) statement that the person "actually selects positive and constructive pathways" (p. 127) contradicts much of human experience outside of the pristine environment of client-centered therapy. Many persons suffer from psychological disturbances. Newspapers report political oppression, acts of human cruelty, and many forms of abuse of people by other people. Evidence everywhere suggests that humans express a mixture of positive and negative tendencies.

The idea of a mixture of positive and negative inherent motives does not address how motives may be integrated. It does not account for why one motive becomes dominant at a particular time. Actualization theory, in contrast, provides a theoretical structure to account for positive and negative behavior. Motivation is singular and inherently constructive from the organism's perspective. Variations in outcome are the result of circumstances that are favorable or unfavorable in respect to persons' specific natures.

The constructive directional definition of the actualization tendency concept results in confusion with a moral or ethical position. A moral or ethical position is also attributed to Rogers when he observes that persons make positive and constructive pathways under the conditions of client-centered therapy. The meaning of constructive at the organismic level refers to the actualization motivational direction towards maintenance, wholeness and realization of potentialities. It does not refer to goodness of an organism's actualization solutions in response to its circumstances, from an ethical or moral perspective. Rogers has been misunderstood as having a moral view of human nature. May (1982), for example, criticized and ridiculed Rogers imputing to him a "good" view of human nature. Rogers' view of the positive actualization tendency, however, did not mean he believed humanity is good. He (1987) wrote:

I have found that if you get to the core of the individual, you discover something constructive, not destructive. People say to me, "Oh, then you believe man is good." I do not like the term **good**. That is a moral judgment....We look at a plant. We do not decide that it is [good or] evil by nature. We just take it for granted that, given the right conditions, it will grow, it will blossom, it will produce its normal life. We do not think that way about humans....I have certainly dealt with plenty of people who are doing evil things, who are doing things that are socially destructive. But,...if you can get to know the person inside, you will find that the person would like to live in harmony and is constructive by nature. And that is the essential basis of the whole theory. (p. 41)

In other words, the actualization tendency is a natural science concept. It should not be interpreted as a moral or ethical idea. The misunderstanding was a source of distress to Rogers. He (1958) wrote:

It disturbs me to be thought of as an optimist. My whole professional experience has been with the dark and often sordid side of life, and I know...the incredibly destructive behavior of which man is capable. (p. 27)

In the context of therapy, clients' constructive choices reveal their prosocial capabilities. These biological innate potentialities are brought out by the facilitative therapeutic conditions. Rogers (1958) wrote:

Man, when you know him deeply, in his worst and most troubled states, is not evil or demonic....We do not need to ask who will socialize him, for one of his deepest needs is for affiliation and communication with others....When we are able to free the individual from defensiveness, so that he is open to the wide range of his own needs, as well as the wide range of environmental and social demands, his reactions may be trusted to be positive, forward-moving, constructive. (p.28)

Pro-social potentialities are part of innate human makeup. They are biological.

One meaning of constructive choice in therapy, however, is ethical. Therapy is partly concerned with the moral or ethical aspects of client's therapeutic movement. A therapy that typically resulted in anti-social and self-destructive outcomes for clients would not be acceptable to clients, therapists or society. This ethical or moral aspect of therapeutic efficacy, however, does not mean that the actualization concept is ethical or moral.

Human innate pro-social characteristics brought out by client-centered therapy are a biological reality. We value those characteristics in ethical terms. But they are biological characteristics. Given pro-social human potentialities, therapy has pro-social results. This is because the actualization tendency motivates the development of potentials. And because the therapy constitutes highly favorable circumstances for persons. The actualization tendency works to fulfill potentials and to develop capabilities that are themselves favorable to the survival of the individual (and, indirectly, to species survival). The actualization tendency has many paths within the person. And it is a natural science concept not a moral or an ethical concept.

The Heuristic Value of the Actualizing Concept

What does actualization theory explain? The actualization tendency is directional and constructive, but it does not necessarily result in positive or constructive outcomes. Human behavior may be constructive or destructive. All possibilities represent outcomes of the actualization tendency. In truth, actualization theory does not explain anything specific. It is a very general set of ideas that help investigators proceed towards specific explanations. The concept of an actualization tendency, like Goldstein's drive to self-actualization, describes the most general characteristic of organismic functioning. It has the value of a general truth that has many implications. It has value because it functions heuristically. The concept functions as a guide to inquiry. It also influences attitudes.

The actualization tendency principle is a particular and fruitful kind of guide to the study of behavior. It is especially helpful if the behavior is unusual or socially unacceptable and if therapies or social solutions are needed. The actualization concept avoids the common mistake of judgementalism. It also avoids invoking religious principles of evil in explaining destructive behavior. Evil may be a valid moral description of certain human behaviors, but it is a dead end as a guide to scientific understanding. Instead, the actualization tendency assumption leads to a particular intellectual and attitudinal approach in understanding those actions. The approach is expressed in the way questions are asked of the phenomena.

A person engages in some form of unconstructive or destructive behavior. Inquiry starts with the assumption of the actualization tendency. A person is necessarily actualizing her nature as best she can under her circumstances. The general question is—how is the person's actualization motivation expressed in this destructive behavior? What are the internal or external circumstances that distort outcomes of the person's inherently constructive directions? How is the destructive behavior serving the maintenance, or the integration, or the fulfillment of the person?

The specific answers depend upon the specific person and situations. But the answers will be ones that make sense of the behavior as an expression of the actualization tendency because the questions are asked from that framework. Answers following from inquiry based on the actualization assumption tend to make sense of destructive behavior in humane terms. Such terms tend to promote compassion and rational considerations. Compassion and rational considerations are fruitful conditions for creative and humane solutions to human problems.

An example of the application of actualization theory can be found in a familiar social-psychological analysis of anti-social gang behavior. Some socially unacceptable behavior may function to enhance social status in certain subcultures. Thus a person's sense of self-value or self-esteem may be enhanced by behavior that is undesirable from the perspective of the larger society. Phenomenologically, the person is engaged in constructive activity.

The enhancement of self-esteem, of course, is not the only possible explanation within actualization theory for gang participation. A person's inner and outer circumstances are studied to discover how the gang became a setting for personal realization. With this approach, gang behavior becomes a comprehensible expression of the actualization tendency. It leads to explanations that reveal how the specific behaviors are aimed toward a personally constructive goal. How does the participant in the gang perceive his whole situation? What are the forces acting upon the person? The theory leads to a pursuit of the function of behavior in terms of how it preserves the person, preserves the person's wholeness, or how it is an expression of further development or realization of capabilities.

The Actualization Tendency's Influence on Attitudes

Actualization theory views persons as functioning as well as they can, under their circumstances at a particular time. They may be able to function better if certain conditions are changed. If unfavorable circumstances can be removed and if favorable circumstances can be created. But, at a given moment, they are doing the best they can. The theory of the actualizing tendency may function in a practitioner's mind as a belief or a hypothesis. Adopted in either form, it is likely to influence attitudes. The helping attitudes that most likely emerge are trust and respect. Trust in persons' capacities to find constructive solutions to their problems and to change their behavior. Respect for persons regardless of their flaws, mistakes or crimes.

The person who adopts the actualizing tendency as a first principle in his or her view of human functioning is likely to hold a compassionate attitude towards people and their shortcomings. Actualization theory implies that people are profoundly innocent. Innate human tendencies are constructive. Destructive feelings and actions must be the result of historical or immediate unfavorable circumstances acting in or on the person. Circumstances are, by definition in the theory, beyond the person's choice or control at that time. The actualization tendency concept implies that people are in a deep sense innocent. Innocent even when they are obviously guilty of bad behavior.

The view that people are inherently innocent promotes understanding and sympathy. It does not preclude moral, ethical or legal judgements about bad behavior. It does not prevent people or social groups from acting rationally to protect themselves or others from persons who commit bad actions. It does not preclude the creation of social consequences for behavior that causes injury to others. It does affect the manner of judgments and the kinds of consequences. It imbues those responses with some degree of compassion.

Another attitude that is shaped by belief in, or by hypothesizing, the actualization tendency is an attitude of facilitation in helping situations. If persons have inherent constructive capabilities, then one would wish to provide circumstances that foster those capabilities. This is a different attitude than wanting to inject or force constructive ideas or practices into other persons. The idea that circumstances distort the results of the actualizing tendency leads to helping methods that facilitate inherent potentialities.

Another attitude that is promoted by belief in, or by hypothesizing, the actualization tendency is a nondirective attitude. The potency and constructive direction of the actualizing motivation fosters the attitude of respect for the person and for the person's innate capacities for self-determination, for finding solutions and for therapeutic change. The helper is motivated to protect the self-determination and autonomy of the person being helped. The helper wants to be careful to not try to control or in any way disempower the person being helped. A nondirective attitude, together with compassion and a facilitative attitude, result in a humane non-authoritarian approach in helping relationships or other human relations situations.

The Actualizing Tendency and Client-Centered Therapy

It is true of all innate characteristics—the more favorable the circumstances, the stronger and more appropriate the expression of the characteristic. Circumstances include the social environment and the internal psychological environment in humans. The latter may involve innate propensities as well as learned attitudes, beliefs, expectations and the characteristics of the individual's self-concept. Thus, in human persons, the pro-social capacities of empathy, affiliation, etc. tend to result in constructive social behavior under adequate or favorable conditions.

Client-centered therapy was created and evolved pragmatically. Rogers' methods and the theory that explained his approach developed because they worked. Clients experienced and displayed therapeutic change that was shown to last (Rogers & Dymond, 1954). As Rogers' therapeutic methods evolved, he formulated theory (Rogers, 1942; 1951; 1957; 1959; 1961; 1977; 1980) and the actualizing tendency concept became more salient in the theory. The basic characteristics of client-centered therapy were pragmatically created. Nevertheless, it is possible to deduce certain features of client-centered therapy from the concept of the actualizing tendency.

Actualization theory posits an idea of an inherent motivation. This motivation is a kind of wisdom of the organism, to persist, to maintain its organization, to heal if needed and to develop its capacities. Favorable circumstances promote specific survival, integrative and developmental processes. Any therapy consequently, should be designed to facilitate relevant developmental processes. At the same time therapy should avoid creating circumstances that undermine or block the processes. The therapeutic attitudes—congruence, unconditional positive regard and empathic understanding—facilitate personal development. Principles of respect and trust and the nondirective attitude protect constructive tendencies. These are logical implications of the actualizing tendency. All together, these salient features of client-centered therapy contribute to its therapeutic potency.

Conclusion

Two fundamental beliefs characterize client-centered therapy. (1) The therapist can trust the client's tendency to grow, develop and heal. (2) All of the therapist's actions must express respect for the client. The respect is for the client as a person who is capable of self-determination, and as a person with capacities for self-understanding and constructive change. These beliefs function as the therapist's fundamental attitudes towards clients. The actualizing tendency concept provides the intellectual grounding for these two functional beliefs. In this way the actualizing tendency has a functional role in client-centered therapy practice (Bozarth & Brodley, 1991).

Rogers' client-centered interpersonal climate taps into human nature and brings out certain human capabilities. It does not bring out others. Client-centered work does not usually bring out the person's gagging and vomiting capability. Less metaphorically, the actualizing tendency motivates persons to realize their more pro-social characteristics. It motivates capabilities for empathy, for protective impulses toward those who are vulnerable. It motivates affiliative tendencies. All of these tendencies are likely to become expressed when the therapy conditions include interpersonal acceptance, empathic understanding and authenticity without the operation of goals or controlling intentions towards the client. The client-centered therapist creates an interpersonal climate that facilitates the potency of the person's inherent actualizing tendency.

Psychotherapy is a moral enterprise (Grant, 1985; Szasz, 1978). "It is an activity which can and does affect the well-being of others, and which is based on ideas about right and wrong in human relationships (Grant, 1990, pp. 79-80)." As much as therapy is a moral or ethical endeavor, it also must be based on the actual nature of human beings in order to be effective. Some practitioners might well proceed as client-centered therapists because the attitudes and behaviors of the therapy seem ethically right to them (as well as being effective). Proceeding on ethical grounds, however, does not deny the naturalistic basis of the therapy's efficacy—a certain human biological nature.

The concept of the actualizing tendency, a concept in the realm of natural science, logically leads a therapist to have a commitment to trust and respect clients. It leads a therapist to maintain a nondirective attitude and to the belief that favorable interpersonal circumstances—embodied in the therapeutic attitudes—can free a person's capacities for health and growth. The actualizing tendency is a premise that is tested each time a therapist chooses to proceed from client-centered theory.

11/98 Published in **A Pessoa Como Centro**, No. 2, 1998, in Portuguese. Used with the permission of the author.

Barbara Temaner Brodley, Ph.D., Illinois School of Professional Psychology—Chicago
Chicago Counseling and Psychotherapy Center

References

Bozarth, J. D. & Brodley, B. T. (1991). Actualization: A functional concept in client-centered therapy. In A. Jones and R. Crandall, (Eds.), **Handbook of self-actualization**. [Special Issue] **Journal of Social Behavior and Personality, 6**(5), 45-59.

Cartwright, D. S. (1957). Annotated bibliography of research and theory construction in client-centered therapy. **Journal of Counseling Psychology, 4**(l), pp. 82-100.

Goldstein, K. (1939). **The organism.** Boston: American Book Company.

Goldstein, K. (1940). **Human nature in the light of psychopathology.** Cambridge: Harvard University Press.

Grant, B. (1985). The moral nature of psychotherapy. **Counseling and Values, 29**(2), 141-150.

Grant, B. (1990). Principled and instrumental nondirectiveness in person-centered and client-centered therapy. **Person-Centered Review, 5**(1), 77-88.

Maslow, A. H. (1970). **Motivation and personality** (2nd ed.). New York: Harper & Row.

May, R. (1982). The problem of evil: An open letter to Carl Rogers. 10-21.

Patterson, C. H. (1984). Empathy, warmth, and genuineness in psychotherapy: A review of reviews. **Psychotherapy, 21**(4), 431-438.

Rogers, C. R. (1942). **Counseling and psychotherapy.** Boston: Houghton Mifflin.

Rogers, C. R. (1951). **Client-centered therapy.** Boston: Houghton Mifflin.

Rogers, C. R. (1954). **Psychotherapy and personality change.** Chicago: University of Chicago Press.

Rogers, C. R. (1957). The necessary and sufficient conditions of therapeutic personality change. **Journal of Consulting Psychology, 21,** 95-103.

Rogers, C. R. (1958). Reinhold Niebuhr's The self and the dramas of history: *A* criticism [with discussion by critics and Rogers' Concluding Comment]. **Pastoral Psychology,** 9(85), 15-28. (Originally published 1956)

Rogers, C. R. (1959). A theory of therapy, personality, and interpersonal relationships as developed in the client-centered framework. In S. Koch (Ed.) **A study of a science: Study I. Conceptual and systematic: Vol. 3 Formulations of the person and the social context** (pp. 184-256). New York: McGraw Hill.

Rogers, C. R. (1961). **Becoming a person.** Boston: Houghton Mifflin.

Rogers, C. R. (1963). The actualizing tendency in relation to "motive" and to consciousness. In M. Jones (Ed.), **Nebraska Symposium on Motivation** (pp. 1-24). U. of Nebraska Press.

Rogers, C. R. (1977). **Carl Rogers on personal power.** New York: Delacorte Press.

Rogers, C. R. (1980). **A way of being.** Boston: Houghton Mifflin.

Rogers, C. R. (1982). Reply to Rollo May's letter. **Journal of Humanistic Psychology, 22,** 85-89.

Rogers, C. R. (1986a). Rogers, Kohut, and Erickson. **Person-Centered Review,** 1(2), 125-140.

Rogers, C. R. (1986b). Client-centered approach to therapy. In I. L. Kutash and A. Wolf (Eds.), **Psychotherapist's casebook: Theory and technique in practice** (pp. 197-208). San Francisco: Jossey Bass.

Rogers, C. R. (1989). Rollo May. In H. Kirschenbaum and V. L. Henderson (Eds.), **Carl Rogers: Dialogues** (pp. 229-255). Boston: Houghton Mifflin.

Rogers, C. R. & Sanford, R. (1984). Client-centered psychotherapy. In H. I. Kaplan and B. J. Sadock (Eds.), **Comprehensive textbook of psychiatry IV** (pp. 1374-1388. Baltimore: Williams & Wilkins.

Szasz, T. (1978). **The myth of psychotherapy.** Garden City, NY: Anchor Press.

Stubbs, J. P. & Bozarth, J. D. (1994). The Dodo bird revisited: A qualitative study of psychotherapy efficacy in research (Special issue). **Journal of Applied and Preventative Psychology**, 3, 109-120.

Thwarting Self-Actualization or Fostering Self-Deactualization: A Person-Centered Perspective

Doug Bower

Carl Rogers (1957, 1961, 1980) presented his case for the "necessary and sufficient conditions" for therapeutic growth. He argued that empathy, congruence, and unconditional positive regard would open the door to the process of self-actualization which is inherent in every person—yea, even in a universal sense, actualization means the forces which enable every aspect of the universe to be in existence.

Basic Assumptions

Self-Actualization

Rogers held that self-actualization is the basis of human potential. Human beings have vast resources for growth and development. Among these resources are the resources for self-understanding, the alteration of the self, and the ability to be self-directive.

We are talking here about the tendency of the organism to maintain itself—to assimilate food, to behave defensively in the face of threat, to achieve the goal of self-maintenance even when the usual pathway to that goal is blocked. We are speaking of the tendency of the organism to move...in the direction of greater independence...Its movement...is in the direction of an increasing self-government, self-regulation, and autonomy, and away from heteronymous control, or control by external forces. (Rogers, 1951, p. 488)

My own argument is that self-actualization is the composite of bio-chemical, physiological, and psychosocial forces or energies which work together to make the self actual or real. These forces are the basis of the existence of a human being who is a self, a person.

While many natural forces come together to form other living entities, some very similar to the human being, the uniqueness of the human being exists as a self. This self can run the gamut of human existence. It's manifestations rest from the primitive peoples of the jungles of South American, to the affluent of Beverly Hills, CA. It's range of manifestations also includes the severely retarded, the psychotic, or the brain damaged who cannot care for themselves and the likes of Albert Einstein, Williams Shakespeare, or Camille Saint Saens.

What is a self? Rogers (1959) explains. It is associated with "Concept of Self," and "Self-structure" which together refer to the organized, consistent gestalt composed of perceptions of the characteristics of the 'I' or 'me' and the perceptions of the relationships of the 'I' or 'me' to others and to various aspects of life, together with the values of the these perceptions. It is a gestalt which is available to awareness though not necessarily in awareness. It is a fluid and changing gestalt, a process, but at any given moment is a specific entity.... (p. 200)

Thwarting Self Actualization

According to Rogers (1958, 1989) the human being is inherently good, not evil.

Yet, if human beings have within them, as Rogers claims, vast, resources for personal growth, why is there crime, hatred, and war? Why do people die? (I won't try to answer the issue of dying). Rogers (1961) was not naive. He was aware of the "incredibly cruel, horribly destructive, immature, regressive, antisocial, hurtful" (p. 27) behaviors evident in human nature. Rogers argued that self actualization can be thwarted.

"The actualization tendency can, of course, be thwarted or warped, but it cannot be destroyed without destroying the organism" (p. 118).

My argument is that when self-actualization is thwarted, persons are stifled, subdued, and oppressed. Creativity is affected and certainly the ability to relate to self and others is greatly infringed upon.

The causes for this thwarting include genetic deformities, microorganisms, society, and psychological forces, perhaps even personal choices as the result of personal experimentation.

Ultimately, I have room for self-deactualization. Lest this sound like we have total control over this, keep in mind that I stated above their are multiple forces which make it possible for a self to exist and/or fail to exist. Stated simply, we come into being and are threatened by nonbeing (Tillich, 1951, 1957). We fall into existence and we fall out of existence. We actualize, and then we deactualize.

I write the last sentence with tentativeness, however. It cannot be said with certainty that we actually fail to exist (deactualize) once we have come into existence (actualize). The Christian tradition alone holds up proclamations concerning eternal life (Or damnation, if you are into that sort of thing). The Holy Scripture of this tradition testifies to a resurrected living Jesus, not merely a martyr. I do not know enough of other religious traditions concerning this issue to comment on them. What little I have seen indicates that other religions have held to a concept or belief that the human being exists in an "after-life."

In addition, modern medicine with its advances in C.P.R. and medical techniques is reporting incidents of "near death experiences." Gabbard & Twemlow (1984), Kung (1994), Kelsey (1982) and others report with optimism and skepticism the tales of persons who have something to say about their personal encounter with "near death." So, while it is clear that human physical bodies cease to function as breathing, heart beating creatures, there may not be absolute self-deactualization.

The focus of this chapter is not upon the extreme form of deactualization (death). It is upon the thwarting of human potential which shall be called for contemplation, deactualization or the thwarting of self-actualization. This deactualization may take mild forms such as defensiveness, insecurity, or mental blocks. It may take on severe forms as psychosis, or violent behavior.

Deactualization

My presupposition is that human beings have interactions with their environment that, at times, inhibit or thwart self-actualization. I know little technical knowledge about genetics and will not address how one's own genetic make-up might contribute to deactualization. I do have some experience with psychosocial phenomena and it is the thwarting of self in this arena upon which I focus the article.

The organism it can be said assembles itself. If that is true, then the organism can disassemble itself. This stepping back into oblivion, and the disassembly of the organism, I can calling deactualization. Yet, on a lessor level, I am arguing that behaviors which emerge preventing the organism to live at its fullest, are the result of self-deactualization.

The Unnecessary and Insufficient Conditions

In 1957, Rogers presented the conditions which helped persons blossom into the self that truly is or can be. "Human nature is basically trustworthy and positive. Individuals can be trusted to act decently and intelligently, given an appropriately facilitative climate" (Natiello, 1994, p. 13). If I say nothing else, Rogers said these conditions were "necessary." That means that they have to be present. Natiello's above statement says that the true person emerges "given an appropriately facilitative climate." This indicates to me that there are climates in which these conditions may not exist at any particular empowering level.

Thus, I am arguing that, if there are conditions which foster the emergence of a self, there are conditions that thwart this self, thus enabling some degree of deactualization.

What are some of these conditions?

Rejection

The first attitude which thwarts self-actualization is rejection. This attitude at best demonstrates conditional regard. "I'll be kind to you only if…." The life situation is negative and restrictions are placed on the subordinates in that situation. Confusion, anger, love, and joy may be oppressed in this unaccepting environment. Further, there are elements of possessiveness and codependency. At its worst, rejection takes the form of abandonment, abuse, even violence or worse. It manifest itself in a severe sense like the ultimate rejection of the likes of Bahaullah, Jesus Christ, Ghandi, Martin Luther King Jr., or John F. Kennedy. Somewhere in the middle of acceptance and severe rejection are cutting comments like, "You're not good enough," and, "You are not wanted here."

On a daily basis, I suppose that rejection can take the form of being denied one's wishes. For instance, a child says to a parent, "I want to go outside and play. I'm bored." The parent looks outside. It is sleeting. The thermometer reads 31 degrees Fahrenheit. "I can't let you go out there. I understand you are bored and want to go outside, but you can't go outside in this weather." The child's wishes are rejected.

What if that rejection comes earlier in life, i.e., the unplanned child. The carelessness of a couple caught up in passion. Suddenly, they are confronted with a new life. When born, this unwanted child lives with the animosity and vindictiveness of one or both of the parents.

Or, a crack baby reaches school age. She is one of those who suffers from a learning disability, an attention deficit, and hyperactivity in the classroom. Her behavior is caustic and alienates fellow students who pick on her. She is of mixed race and is frowned upon by classmates and adults. Because of her learning problems she is singled out by the teachers and school officials as one who cannot learn and as a "trouble maker." Her behavioral problems bring her into conflict with the teacher. She feels unliked. She doesn't measure up to the standards of the society in which she is functioning.

"We'll only love you if" is a common theme with rejection. "We'll accept you if you behave just right." "You can come here if you have good grades." "I'll take you out to eat if you are nice to me" (that is translated, "if you do what I want").

Rejection takes the form of conditional regard, aloofness, apathy, disinterest, and/or laissez-faire.

Misunderstanding

A second ingredient for thwarting self-actualization is misunderstanding. Here little effort is made to grasp or sense the feelings and experiences of individuals. This, I suppose, is a form of rejection. There is little appreciation for what is going on inside individuals. Listening to one other is poor in quality and often blocked by efforts to make sure that everyone adheres to a certain set of beliefs or experiences. For instance, during family discussions the youngest or weakest member of the family is told to shut-up when the parents or strongest members of the family are talking. Eventually, the child ambers around the room and soon is "getting into things" and conflict arises with the parents. Punishment results in spankings, or isolation from the family. There is little understanding or tolerance of curiosity and exploration.

For a adolescent "getting into things" might mean getting into trouble with the law, fights at school, sexual promiscuity, or any number of "things."

A couple goes for counseling. The husband says he wants to grow. He feels he yells too much. The wife has had enough and wants out of the relationship. They fight, they scold, they yell at each other over "silly things." They don't hear each others' concerns because they are too intent on making each other understand. "I don't feel understood" and "Nobody ever listens to me" are common complaints.

Incongruence

A third condition which thwarts self-actualization and promotes deactualization is incongruence. I characterizing incongruence insecurity, insincerity, deceitfulness, instability.

Individuals in this state often feel like they are not themselves. They put up fronts and facades out of anxiety and concern that they will really not be appreciated for who they really are. Their experiences tend not to be available to awareness. They are closed to their feelings and others complain that they are difficult to get to know.

A young woman complains that she never does the things she wants to do. Her husband and children get what they want. Even when she is sick, she waits on the family and takes care of their needs. Inside she harbors resentment. Her husband comes and goes as he pleases. She can't even take a walk without getting "fussed at." However, she also readily admits that she tends not to tell anybody what she wants until she explodes in a furious tantrum of screaming and yelling. "I don't know what I want' and "I don't know what to say" are common statements for the incongruent person.

The Thwarted Self and Its Manifestations

Incongruence breeds incongruence. Bower (1985) described incongruence as a state of discrepancy existing between the self that is, and the self-concept. "When a person is incongruent, there is a difference between the experiences which comprise the actual self and the perceptions of those self experiences" (p. 52).

In this state, feelings and experiences are denied to awareness. They are too dangerous, too unwanted. Punishment and put-downs might very well result when the true self emerges.

Thus "the individual perceives his experiences selectively, in terms of the conditions of worth which have come to exist in him" (Rogers, 1959, p. 226).

Anxiety

If the self is perceived as dangerous, and if that self is throttled, when it begins to emerge, inner conflict between the self and the self-concept results. The individual wants to ask for something, but the tension mounts. A fear-like condition predominates. His or her hands may shake and a cold sweat may develop. A sense of impending doom may prevail, but there may seem to be no enemy to fear. These individuals may not even know why they feel the way they do. They may only know that under certain circumstance they feel the misery of anxiety.

Further Signs of a Thwarted Self

The thwarted self if a suppressed self. Here the individual "keeps a lid on" feelings and experiences. Thus one's experience is withheld from one's self and others.

The thwarted self is inaccessible. Feelings, and experiences are often denied access to awareness or consciousness. "I don't know what I feel" is a common remark. Since the person doesn't admit the feelings and experiences to awareness, he/she can't share them with others either.

The thwarted self is a rigid self. This person has trouble adjusting to change. The acceptance of any changes becomes difficult as the person hangs on to long held patterns of behavior.

The thwarted self is blocked. If I won't admit feelings and experiences to awareness, then it make sense that my life seems all right at the level of awareness. I have no troubles. Everyone else has problems, not me.

The thwarted self is legalistic. The person's life is full of "oughts" and "shoulds" or the opposite. "I should feel guilty for being angry at my mother." "I ought to be nice to my brother and sister."

The legalist self is one which spends a great deal of energy meeting the expectations of others. The individual goes to a college chosen by his father. She becomes a housewife, because of pressures from family members. "I never seem to do or go what I want. You always get your way." In pleasing others, the person stuffs or blocks thoughts and feelings, and others fail to know there is a problem. Even if the thoughts and experiences are shared, the reactions of others seem so overwhelming that it is best to keep quiet. "If you can't say anything nice, don't say anything at all."

The legalist self also expects others to live similar lifestyles to his or her own. We dress similarly, think similarly, eat the same kinds of foods. We "ought" to vote the same as well.

The thwarted self is simplistic, narrow minded, and thus bigoted. There is no grappling with issues and problems. "There is only one way to heaven, and we (Catholics, Baptists, Methodists, etc.) are the only ones going there." "Niggers are all alike. I can't even tell them a part. They're slow and stupid." Issues, problems, and their solutions are either "black or white." There are no compromises.

The thwarted self feels inadequate. This individual has been told all his or her life that he or she is not good enough. Not surprisingly, this person has difficulty accepting praise and thanks for action that is appreciated. Thus, there is a chronic sense of never being good enough.

The thwarted self is a rejecting self. Since I'm not good enough, no one else is either. Your statements, your papers, your thoughts, your ideas, your choices, your dreams, your behavior, etc. are not good enough. You haven't reached your potential. Every effort that belongs to you is rejected and put down.

The thwarted self is distrustful. "You are up to something." "You're just trying to get me to do what you want." "You must be cheating on me." This person cannot give love and care to others or may not be able to accept care from others. "Watch out, I'll only get hurt any way.

She'll leave me once she finds out who I really am."

The thwarted self is alienated. This state of alienation is the feeling of isolation from others. The individual feels that there are no friends, family, or colleagues on whom to call for help. "They wouldn't be interested in my problem and I wouldn't want to burden them." It seems to this person that nobody cares and that no one appreciates him or her. Feelings of loneliness are common.

The thwarted self is negative. "I'll never be able to do that. I can't...." People in this negative state tend to see only the obstacles to change. There is no confidence that the obstacles can be overcome.

The thwarted self lacks identity. "Who am I. What is my purpose in life." This living, breathing, thinking being cannot grasp personal identity. So, search after search is conducted in an attempt to fine the true self.

The thwarted self maintains facades. The line from a hit song of years gone by "Smiling faces tell lies" reflects facades. "I laugh to keep from crying." How many times have therapists seen clients who bitterly complained that they put up fronts to their parents, or significant others only to feel miserable for not expressing or asserting themselves.

All human beings experience the thwarting of the self to some degree or another. On rare occasions, during religious moments, peak experiences, times of tremendous creativity, we get a glimpse of the self that truly is. Most of the time we battle with forces within and without that oppress the self and keep it from blooming into a beautiful flower.

I liken this to a war of psychological powers and principalities. The old good versus evil stuff.

An Optimistic Paradigm

Rogers (1961) offers some of the characteristics of this thwarted self as he or she begins therapy.

There is an unwillingness to communicate self....

Feelings and person meanings are neither recognized nor owned....

Personal constructs...are extremely rigid.

Close and communicative relationships are construed and dangerous.

No problems are recognized or perceived....

There is no desire to change.

There is much blockage of internal communication. (p. 132)

Rogers believed that the doors to the process of self-actualization could be opened under the right conditions, the conditions of empathy, unconditional positive regard, and congruence. If the door was opened a wonderfully complex, creative, resourceful human being would be discovered and liberated.

The goal of the collaborative therapeutic relationship is always the growth/healing of the client, although the collaborative effort tends to increase the satisfaction and personal effectiveness of client and therapist by generating increased energy, empowerment, creativity, openness, and receptivity. (Natiello, 1994, p. 11)

The Self-Actualizing or Fully Functioning Person

What are the characteristics of self-actualizing people which emerge as the result of living in environments rich in the "necessary and sufficient conditions." Maslow (1968, 1971) believed that numerous characteristics can be noted in self-actualizing people including: a realistic orientation; acceptance of self, others and life situations; spontaneity; autonomy and independence; unstereotyped impressions of others; profound mystical and spiritual experiences; identification with humankind; profound and deep intimate relationships; democratic values and attitudes; a philosophical sense of humor; creativeness; and transcendence of the environment (Hall & Lindzey, 1978).

Rogers (1961) presented five stages to therapy in which the therapeutic conditions were present over an unstated period of time. In the fifth stage, presumably a stage marking the process of therapeutic growth, Rogers presented nine evident qualities. 1) The free expression of feelings in the present. 2) These feelings are nearly "fully experienced." 3) A tendency to realize that the experience of feelings lies within the client rather than outside of the client. 4) The client experiences "surprise and fright" in relationship to feelings that emerge. 5) There is a tendency toward ownership of one's feelings. 6) Experiencing tends to move more toward the here-and-now with little postponement. 7) There are more new personal discoveries with self examination and questioning of those discoveries. 8) There is movement toward precision in capturing the essence of feelings and their meanings. 9) There is tendency to confront the contradictions and incongruences of self experiences. 10) There is acceptance of self-responsibility and a sense of one's participation in personal situations and experiences.

Rogers (1963) summarized three facets to the person who emerged from successful therapy. 1) There would be an openness to experience. 2) A living in an existential mode

("Each moment would be new...the self...would emerge from experience, rather than experience being translated or twisted to fit a preconceived self-structure" p. 20). 3) The person would feel competent and trustworthy concerning his/her behavior. This person is able to live fully in and all of his feelings and reactions. He is making use of all his organic equipment to sense, as accurately as possible, the existential situation within and without. He is using all of the data his nervous system can thus supply, using it in awareness. He is able to permit his total organism to function in all its complexity in selecting, from the multitude of possibilities, that behavior which in this moment of time will be most generally and genuinely satisfying. He is able to trust his organism in this functioning, not because it is infallible, but because he can be fully open to the consequences of each of his actions and correct them if they prove to be less than satisfying.

He is able to experience all of his feelings, and is afraid of none of his feelings; he is his own sifter of evidence, but is open to evidence from all sources; he is completely engaged in the process of being and becoming himself, and thus discovers that he is soundly and realistic social, he lives completely in this moment, but learns that this is the soundest living for all time. He is a fully functioning organism, and because of the awareness of himself which flows freely in and through his experiences, he is a fully functioning person. (pp. 21-22)

Conclusion

At the risk of being simplistic, I have prepared a line diagram.

Rejection   Acceptance
Misunderstanding   Empathy
Incongruence   Congruence
--------------------------(Self)------------------------
Psychosis   Fully
Violent Behavior   Functioning
Etc.   Person

CeN   Figure 1

At one extreme, on the left, I have placed rejection, misunderstanding, and incongruence. Below it I have placed examples of human behaviors which I believe to be related to these conditions.

At the other end, on the right, I have placed acceptance, empathy, and congruence. Below them I have placed Rogers' (1963) term of the Fully Function Person. The line represents the self. At one end, the self is thwarted and manifests itself in destructive ways. On the other end, the self flows and manifests itself in creative, resourceful kinds of ways. Still, even on the left hand side, something of the resourcefulness and creativeness of the human being manifests itself. Even in the midst of a severely restrictive environment the potato (Rogers, 1980) sends out its roots striving for nourishment to survive. So it is with the human being. The self seeks to emerge and prevail.

Self-Actualization can be thwarted. The conditions which foster self-deactualization include rejection, incongruence, and misunderstanding. The thwarted self is manifested in a variety of forms such as anxiety, rigidity, distrust, alienation, legalism and others.

The self-actualizing person conversely has a variety of available experiences such as openness to self and others, acceptance, autonomy, spontaneity, etc.

References

Bower, D. W. (1985). **Assumptions and attitudes of the Rogerian person-centered approach to counseling: Implications for pastoral counseling**. Unpublished master's project, Columbia Theological Seminary, Decatur, GA.

Gabbard, G. O., & Twemblow, S. W. (1984). **With the eyes of the mind: An empirical analysis of out-of-body states**. New York: Praeger.

Hall, C. S., & Gardner, L. (1978). **Theories of personality** (3rd ed.). New York: John Wiley & Sons.

Kelsey, M. (1982). **Afterlife: The other side of dying**. New York: Crossroad.

Kung, H. (1984). **Eternal life? Life after death as a medical, philosophical, and theological problem** (L. Quinn, Trans.). New York: Doubleday.

Maslow, A.H. (1968). **Toward a psychology of being** (2nd ed.). New York: Van Nostrand Reinhold Company.

Maslow, A.H. (1971). **The farther reaches of human nature**. New York: The Viking Press.

Natiello, P (1994). The collaborative relationship in psychotherapy. **The Person-Centered Journal**, 1 (2), 11-17.

Rogers, C. R. (1957). The necessary and sufficient conditions of therapeutic personality change **Journal of Consulting Psychology**, 21, 95-103.

Rogers, C. R. (1958). Reinhold Niebuhr's The self and the dramas of history: *A* criticism [with discussion by critics and Rogers' Concluding Comment]. **Pastoral Psychology**, 9(85), 15-28. (Originally published 1956)

Rogers, C. R. (1959). A theory of therapy, personality, and interpersonal relationships, as developed in the client-centered framework. In S. Koch (Ed.), **Psychology: A study of a science**, Vol. III. **Formulations of the person and the social context**. New York: McGraw-Hill, pp. 184-256.

Rogers, C. R. (1963). **On becoming a person**. Boston: Houghton Mifflin.

Rogers, C. R. (1963). The concept of the fully functioning person. **Psychotherapy: Theory, Research and Practice, 1**, 17-26.

Rogers, C. R. (1980). **A way of being**. Boston: Houghton Mifflin.

Rogers, C. R. (1989). Notes on Rollo May. In H. Kirshenbaum, & V. L. Henderson (Eds.) **Carl Rogers: Dialogues**. Boston: Houghton Mifflin, pp. 237-239.

Tillich, P. (1951). **Systematic theology** (Vol. 1). Chicago: The University of Chicago Press.

Tillich, P. (1957). **Systematic theology** (Vol. 2). Chicago: The University of Chicago Press.

Toward a Philosophy of Person-Centered Therapeutic Growth: Using a Basic Understanding of the Process Theory of Alfred North Whitehead

Doug Bower

The foundational presupposition of the person-centered approach to therapy is that under the "necessary and sufficient conditions" (Rogers, 1957), personal growth and restructuring of the self can occur. It is also basic to the approach that if the "necessary and sufficient conditions" are present, the client, the therapist and others will experience those conditions (Rogers, 1957). This is not to say that experiencing is always a conscious process whereby there is profound awareness of the conditions. My own experience with clients has been that even though I felt I maintained high levels of the core conditions, clients don't always have an awareness. I have also experienced times in which I did a poor job of maintaining the core conditions, but the client reported feeling accepted, and understood and that I was genuine.

This chapter presents a philosophical basis for the experiencing of the "conditions" and the experience of change using the "process" theory of Alfred North Whitehead (1929). It is a well known position of person-centered theory that the attitudinal qualities of empathy, unconditional positive regard and congruence of person-centered therapists cannot be discovered unless the therapist is encountered and thus experienced

(Rogers, 1957). Whitehead's (1929) theory of process and reality supplies a philosophical basis for the encounter and the experience, conscious or unconscious, that occurs between client and therapist.

Experiencing the Necessary and Sufficient Conditions

Rogers (1957, 1961, 1980) argued that therapeutic growth takes place in relationship to certain attitudinal qualities—empathy, unconditional positive regard and congruence. Rogers (1957, 1961, 1980) believed that these qualities have to be present in the therapist, in the therapeutic relationship and, ideally, perceived by the client.

Rogers (1951) argued that when these conditions are present and observed by the client and when the potential for growth becomes realized, changes are often observable. He presented many observations concerning changes in therapy, including, (a) changes in material presented (e.g., movement from talking about problems to statements of insight), (b) changes in perception and attitude concerning self (e.g., increase in positive self-references), © changes in differentiation of perception (e.g., perceptions of experiences, feelings, self, others and environment), (d) increase in awareness concerning previously denied experiences, (e) changes in valuing (e.g., what is regarded as "good" or "bad" is perceived differently), (f) changes in personality, (g) changes in behavior (e.g., did the client stop abusing his/her children?).

Rogers (1951) also reported that the clients had experiences during therapy. These included (a) discovering responsibility for the self, (b) self-exploration, © uncovering of denied experiences or attitudes, (d) reorganization of the self, (e) a sense of progress, and (f) an experience of the ending of therapy.

Rogers (1961) presented some additional experiences that can occur during therapy. He stated that (a) there is an experiencing of the self, (b) a coming to like one's self, and © a becoming one's own organism or experience. The presence of the "necessary and sufficient conditions" produces a process in which there is a moving away from fixity, remoteness from feelings and experience, rigidity of self-concept, remoteness from people, impersonality of functioning. It moves toward fluidity, changingness, immediacy of feelings and experience, acceptance of feelings and experience, tentativeness of constructs, discovery of a changing self in one's changing experience, realness and looseness of relationships, a unity and integration of functioning. (Rogers, 1961, pp. 64-65)

Again, Rogers (1980) stated that he believed that when persons encountered "the attitudinal qualities," "constructive" and "growthful" changes took place. "Persons in an environment infused with these attitudes develop more self-understanding, more self confidence, more ability to choose their behaviors" (Rogers, 1980, p. 133). Over the years, numerous studies and papers have sought to present the discovery of the impacts of therapeutic relationships under the conditions of empathy, unconditional positive regard and congruence (Bergin & Solomon, 1963; Combs, 1986; Gurman, 1977; Rice, 1983; Seeman, 1954). These studies and papers have added to the belief that the "attitudinal qualities" have made an impact on the lives of many clients. This is not a denial of course that there are studies that disavow the impact of the core conditions. However, disavowing the impact of the core conditions does not produce client-centered therapists.

Basic Foundational Blocks of Whitehead to be Applied in this Chapter

Actual Occasions

The basic unit of Whitehead's (1929) theory is the actual occasion. "'Actual entities'—also termed 'actual occasions'—are the final real things of which the world is made up" (p. 18). The actual occasion is the "pulsating experiencing" and "momentary embodiment" of existence (Jackson, 1981).

Each moment of experiencing…has an identical structure. It begins in the initial phase, grows together through intermediate or supplemental phases, and completes itself in the final phase of "satisfaction." As completed it is a new datum for the next moment of becoming. (Jackson, pp. 3-4)

During the initial phase, a datum from the past is "prehended" and "grasped" in the new moment and becomes a part of the experience of the present moment (Jackson, 1981). There are of course an infinite number of actual occasions which immediately precede each new occasion and an infinite number of parallel occasions to which the past occasions prehend. The most directly associated past occasions and the nearest parallel occasions have the greatest impact.

As the occasion progresses into the intermediate phase, there is an endeavor to gather all the data from the past, from God, and from other occasions of the present, as well as its own "aims" to create a "novel" and "unique" experience (Jackson, 1981). The occasion will "sift many feelings, struggle for depth and harmony, as it is guided by its aim toward what it wills to become" (p. 5).

In the final phase, the moment of experience reaches completeness. The moment is finished. It has achieved its aim. "It is what it is" (p. 5). The occasion now becomes a datum for the future occasion and the cycle repeats itself with new twists provided in the future occasion, from other past occasions and from God. "So actuality comes into being, has its 'moment,' and ceases to experience'" (p. 5). It continues only as an experience in future generations of occasions.

Nexus

The next aspect of Whitehead's (1929) theory is the nexus. The nexus is "a 'relation' between occasions" (p. 194). These occasions share their momentary experience together. "There are an indefinite number of relations realized between the occasions of any particular nexus" (p. 194).

Society

Closely related to the nexus is the society. The society is the personal ordering of a nexus.

A 'society,' in the sense in which that term is here used, is a nexus with social order; and an 'enduring object,' or 'enduring creature,' is a society whose social order has taken the special form of 'personal order.' (Whitehead, 1929, p. 34)

The society or the personal order of the nexus involves a serial relation. Nexus A gives itself to nexus B which in turn prehends the occasions of A, but B adds its own twist of novelty thus making B a unique set of moments of experience similar to but different from any nexus which precedes it or which exists simultaneously with B. The serial continues in C, D, etc., and thus creates the nexus called an "enduring object."

These serials, "societies", form electrons, protons, and other aspects of atoms. As more complex societies are formed, societies become atoms, then molecules. Even more complex societies become inorganic materials or organic organizations called cells. Inorganic materials often are found as elements such as sulfur, gold, or oil. Cells as organic organizations, on the other hand, might reach further complexities as organs, tissues and bodies. The human body and brain are such organic complex society of occasions.

This doctrine, that the true individuals are momentarily experiences, means that what we ordinarily call individuals, the sorts of things that endure through time, are not true individuals, but are "societies" of such. Personal human existence is a "serially ordered society" of occasions of experience. (Cobb & Griffin, 1976, p. 15)

The complex society of occasions is manifest in its cellular composition. Certain occasions form the cells which make up the cardiovascular system. Certain occasions form the cells of the gastrointestinal tract, the muscles, the eyes. And certain occasions form the cells and the unique functions of the brain. All these serial nexi as well as others function together to form the complex society called the human being.

Experiencing Others

Here now is the basis of experiencing another person. The occasions become what they are. The "duration" of the serially ordered societies called the human being "complex society of experiencing occasions" (Jackson, 1981, p. 3). Human beings are thus collections of special types of occasions found in nature which endure a given period of time. Each person offers idiosyncratic twists to what it means to be human while maintaining similarities with each other. They are part of the observational present which is based on preceding occasions, and which will have an impact on the occasions which are yet to be. The occasions of an individual are prehended by the another making novelty and new aims possible in the other.

When the occasions of one human being are prehended by the occasions of another, experiencing takes place. These experiences vary in variety, duration, intensity and impact. It may also vary at the level of awareness and can thus be conscious or unconscious. In the process of experiencing all there is always something novel about these experiences as each occasion and the complex society of occasions presents its own new twists and develops their own new aims for the new ".momentary embodiment" of existence (Jackson, 1981).

Attitudinal Qualities Prehended

Whitehead's (1919, 1929) process theory provides a philosophical basis for why the attitudinal qualities work. When a therapist maintaining the "necessary and sufficient conditions" encounters an incongruent client, the occasions of each are prehended and impacted by each. An impression is made which is experienced and can be observed and described which can provide a rich source of experiences concerning the therapist and the client. The therapist experiences the client, and the client, with his or her own occasions, experiences the therapist and becomes free to change or grow.

An Example

S was a 36 year old female who shot and killed her husband who was in the process of attacking her. Arrested for the murder of her husband, she was later acquitted under the conditions of self-defense. During her time in jail, S began to hallucinate and her language became disjointed and confused. She decompensated.

After her release from jail, S returned to work and began to believe her supervisor called her over the loudspeakers to come up to the office so he could have sex with her. She would also walk down the streets of the town in which she lived and believe by-passers were plotting against her because of what she did to her husband.

Her work suffered and eventually she was discharged from work.

Shortly after being fired, the local police found her wandering the streets talking incoherently. They took her to the local branch of the state mental health unit where she was diagnosed as paranoid schizophrenic but not needing hospitalization.

As her condition deteriorated, her brother became her guardian and executor and eventually her children were placed in foster homes. Still she was not hospitalized.

When I first met her, she had been in the mental health system for about a year. She failed to keep her appointments on a regular basis and did not take her medication as prescribed.

She was a test for my early attempts at empathy. I had just begun my pilgrimage into the person-centered approach and was unconvinced, uncertain and insecure about the "necessary and sufficient conditions," especially empathy.

I found S extremely difficult to understand. To me, her conversation was disjointed and disconnected. As best I could follow, S said her husband had been a pimp. She said people on the streets were plotting against her. She said her supervisor at work used to page her over the intercom to come to his office so he could have sex with her.

Her statements seemed so bizarre to me that I got confused trying to follow her. "How can I be empathic when I don't even understand what the client is saying?" I asked myself.

As I continued to work with S, and continued to put the "attitudinal qualities" to the test through my own adherence to and development of these skills and through my observing S, I found an answer to my question: My experience of the disjointedness, the disconnectedness, the confusion, the bizarreness was the answer. It was the result of being empathic. S was disjointed, disconnected and confused. She was overwhelmed by her own world and was making her attempts to become herself under the adverse conditions in her life.

I found that I prized S and accepted her confusion, disconnectedness and disjointedness. I continued to try to enter her world even though I felt at the time I was failing in that effort.

Over the course of 2 years of working with S, I noticed changes. The changes were subtle sometimes, dangerous and frightening at others. S started coming for therapy more often. At first she came once a month, then every other week, and then every week. She became more coherent. I found that her husband was not a pimp, but that he did sleep around a lot. I found he had been physically abusing her for many years. I also found that she was not far off base about people on the streets plotting against her. She lived in a small town and people knew each other. Many knew she had shot and killed her husband. Many knew she had gone "crazy." Many were afraid of her and probably did talk about her. I did find out, however, that her supervisor never had made any sexual advances to her.

As she changed more and more, she became dangerous and scared her family and friends. one day in a power struggle with her brother over her children and control of the house, she took a gun and shot into the air over his head as a sign warning him not to bother her any more. She wound up in the state hospital for 3 days for that incident. I kept in mind that S's aim could kill and she did not kill. Instead she used the fear others had of her and her gun to frighten. It was very effective. Her brother stopped bothering her and the price she paid was 3 days in the state hospital. Her growth continued and she became less frightening to people. She was given permission by the state to see and be with her children. She was far more coherent and had more control of herself. She had reached a point at which she felt secure enough with herself to reenter the work environment.

Unfortunately, my practicum at the local mental health branch came to an end. I do not know what has happened with S since that time. I did, however, see some changes which had not occurred previously. While I believe strongly in the potential of all individuals (though what that potential is different from individual to individual), I believe that those changes in S occurred in relationship to my maintaining the "attitudinal qualities." I wish that I could say that all the changes I saw were regarded as good by others, but when you get shot at, it is hard to appreciate some changes. As for me, I saw some of S's efforts to become herself directed outwardly. Instead of directing her powerful anger inward, she directed it outwardly. Unfortunately, she used a gun as a means of that expression. I hope that she has found a safer way of expressing that anger without going "crazy" in the process or without using such a negative weapon.

This case illustrates for me, at least, that when the "attitudinal qualities" are present and prehended by another. The new occasions of the therapist and the client make new changes possible. S had become more coherent, more connected in her thinking. She acted more logically I thought. Even the shouting incident made sense to me. I regret she didn't seem to think of a deeper legal way to handle her crisis with her brother, but I do consider what she did a step above shooting and killing someone. I also think she was headed toward more constructive handling of crisis than using a gun to run off her critics.

I don't condone violence. Yet, I have found that in roaming around in the world of another, their behavior, though legally reprehensible, often makes sense.

Discussion

I hope that is clear in this chapter that part of the rationale for the growth of individuals in therapy rests on the impact of the attitudinal qualities of the person-centered therapist upon the client. I am not arguing that change takes place because of behavioral modifications through modeling, tokens or rewards. Neither am I arguing that change takes place simply because the client has innate capacities for change. I am arguing for the necessity of the attitudinal qualities and the prehending of these qualities by the client as resources for change. With the prehension of the attitudinal qualities, new twists to the aims of the occasions which make up the client can be possible. Growth can occur. Indeed, Rogers (1951, 1961, 1980) states that clients report change.

This change can be slow. There are occasions within the client and outside the client's immediate self which have the impact of oppressing growth potential and thwarting the process. Yet as the new occasions of empathy, unconditional positive regard and congruence are prehended by the client and as the client's own novelties begin to emerge, the occasions which bring liberty of self become more numerous and are prehended again and again, and the occasions which are oppressive become less powerful and less impactful. The client becomes freer to grow.

Conclusions

Rogers and his colleagues argued that therapeutic change is possible through the "necessary and sufficient conditions" of empathy, unconditional positive regard, and congruence as maintained and adhered to by the person-centered therapist. Why do the attitudinal qualities work? Whitehead (1929) might say they work because they are prehended by the client and thus offer new data to be used by the client's own occasions. The innate capacity of the client to bring new twists and novelties to his or her own realities are thus enhanced because of the experiences with the therapist, and growth can occur.

References

Bergin, A. E., & Solomon, S. (1963, September). Personality and performance correlates of empathy understanding in psychotherapy. Paper presented at the meeting of the American Psychological Association, Philadelphia.

Combs, A. W. (1986). What makes a good helper? A person-centered approach. **Person-Centered Review**, 1(1), 51-61.

Gurman, A. S. (1977). The patient's perception of the therapeutic relationship. In A. S. Gurman & A. M. Razin (Eds.), **Effective psychotherapy: A handbook of research** (pp. 503-543). Oxford: Pergamon Press.

Jackson, G. E. (1981). **Pastoral care and process theology**. Washington: University Press of America.

Rice, L. N. (1983). The relationship in client-centered therapy. In M. J. Lambert (Ed.), **Psychotherapy and patient relationships** (pp. 36-60). Homewood, IL: Dow Jones-Irwin.

Rogers, C. R. (1951). **Client-centered therapy**. Boston: Houghton Mifflin.

Rogers, C. R. (1957). The necessary and sufficient conditions of therapeutic personality change. **The Journal of Consulting Psychology**, 21, 95-103.

Rogers, C. R. (1961). **On becoming a person**. Boston: Houghton Mifflin.

Rogers, C. R. (1980). **A way of being**. Boston: Houghton Mifflin.

Seeman, J. (1954). Counselor judgments of therapeutic process and outcome. In C. R. Rogers & R. Dymond (Eds.), **Psychotherapy and personality change** (pp. 99-108). Chicago: University of Chicago Press.

Whitehead, A. N. (1919). **Concept of nature**. London: Cambridge University Press.

Whitehead, A. N. (1929). **Process and reality**. New York Macmillan: Free Press.

Features of Person-Centered Therapy

Doug Bower

This is a chapter which emerges from reflections on one particular project (Bower, 1985) that was developed to determine characteristics of the person of a select group of person-centered therapists. The intent of the study was to make inferences concerning the characteristics of the person-centered approach to therapy. A similar project was later completed (Bower, 1989).

Research Philosophy

The investigation was designed to identify characteristics of selected person-centered therapeutic relationships by means of qualitative analysis (Patton, 1980). Qualitative methodology was used as it is designed to minimize preconceptions concerning the subject being investigated (Goetz & LeCompte, 1984). It enables the investigator to assume a position of naivete in order to make fresh discoveries about the subject or object being studied even if it has been investigated many times previously.

This methodology was also chosen to examine of the perceptions of those involved in the study (Goetz & LeCompte, 1984). This intent seems consistent with Rogers' (1957, 1961, 1980) idea of empathy in therapy. This study is based on the effort to enter into the world of the participants "is if...."

An important presupposition brought into this investigation is that every datum that emerges during the investigation is important (Goetz & LeCompte, 1984). This means, in part, that each comment and each observation from the data sources are important whether or not the comment or observation is repeated by other data sources. Any datum is considered to have potential if not real value. Of course, if a datum is observed from differing perspectives, this makes it stronger. This does not mean that every datum will turn out to be relevant for the report, but it does mean that every datum is important and taken seriously.

Method

Preliminary Groundwork

Letters were sent to several person-centered therapists who had studied under Carl Rogers or had been involved in numerous workshops led by Rogers, and who were recognized by the investigator to be known client-centered/person-centered therapists.

The letters requested that the therapist provide an audio tape recording with a client (blank tapes were provided by the investigator). The letters also asked each therapist to respond to a brief questionnaire, and that each client respond to a brief questionnaire. Each therapists was informed that observers would listen to the audio tapes and would present their observations concerning anything they noticed during their listening.

Ten client-centered/person-centered therapists responded to the initial letters, but only six returned materials for analysis. Code numbers were assigned to each therapist who responded to the initial letters.

Procedure

Tapes, questionnaires and release of information forms were sent to the therapists who indicated their willingness to participate in the project.

Data were obtained from the questionnaires received from the therapists and the clients. These data were then coded (Glaser & Strauss, 1967; Goetz & LeCompte, 1984; Strauss, 1987; Strauss & Corbin, 1990).

Three observers, one a person-centered therapist, one an eclectically oriented counselor, and one who was naive about the theory and practice of therapy, listened to each tape. No formal questionnaire was given to the listeners. They were told to simply write down their observations and reactions. Any observation was welcome and encouraged. After listening to a tape, each observer was interviewed so that any ambiguous responses could be clarified.

The data were then coded. Since data were received from three types of resources, therapists, clients and observers, they could automatically be coded easily under each of those categories.

Data from the therapists, the clients and observers were analyzed for evidence of any patterns that might be contained (Patton, 1980).

Categories were organized by data source, listeners' observations, therapists' observations, and clients' observations.

Results

All the relevant data are being reported here. Each category is presented, listeners, therapists, and clients.

Listeners' observations

Analysis of the data from the listeners led to the discovery of three categories: data which related to the person of the therapist, data which related to the therapists' techniques or style, data which consisted of evaluative reactions to the therapy.

Person of the therapist

One therapist was described as "supportive," "nonjudgmental," "promotes expression," "didn't get irritated," "mothering," "helpful," "inviting," "attentive," "patient," and warm."

A second therapist was observed as "enthusiastic," "empathic," "agreeable," "easygoing," "relaxed," "tender," "not surprised," "receptive," "dominating," was "intense," "tuned in" and as one who "listens."

A third therapist was seen as "gentle," "soft," "patient," "spontaneous," "accepting," "nonjudgmental," "interested," "concerned," "dominating at times," "gentle,"and as having an "easy manner." It was also stated that the therapist "moves easily with client."

A fourth therapist was described as "accepting," "friendly," and having a "sense of humor." One listener stated the therapist "disappears" and another said the "client would have continued talking even if she were talking to a brick wall." Yet another observer stated: "I can't tell that the counselor makes a real difference here."

A fifth therapist was seen as "supportive," comfortable," "silent," "sensitive," "warm," "tender," "nonjudgmental," "accepting," "soothing," "curious," "genuine," "real," "invitational," "relaxed," "nonthreatening,""inactive,""responsive," and as having "staying power (patient)."

The last therapist was described as "open," "patient," "nonjudgmental," "tender," "accepting," "kind," "reactive," "responsive," "permitting," and "sharing."

Therapists' techniques or style

The listeners also made observations concerning characteristics of the therapists' techniques or style. The first therapist used "Yes, uh-huh." Other observations of this therapist's style was that it was "nonconfrontive," "reflective," "summarizing," "interruptive," "interpretive," "encouraged the client to bitch," "put a stamp of approval on bitching," "attempted to understand," "focused on feelings," "focused on client," and "mechanical."

Listeners stated that the second therapist "repeats what was said," "clarifies," "explores," uses "reflection," was "interpretive," and often said "Yeah, yeah."

Listeners said that the third therapist "disappeared." Other characteristics regarding this therapist's technique or style included "reflective," "attentive," "interruptive," "clarifying," "confrontive," "active," "speculative,""silence," "summarizes," "asks questions." The it was also noted that the therapist used "Uh-huh, yes" as a response. It was also noted that the therapist "listens" and is "encouraging."

For the fourth therapist, listeners noted the use of "Uh-huh." They also noted that the therapist "laughs," "asks questions," "repeated," "used brief self-disclosure," used "reflection," "summarized," made "comparisons," "encourages continuation," and was "clarifying."

The fifth therapist was seen by listeners as using "silence," "asking questions," engaging in "confrontation," "allowing the client to emote," having "listened," and being "focused."

The characteristics of the last therapist's technique were that the therapist "listens," was "silent," used "clarification," "self-disclosure," "asked questions," "shared observations," "summarized," and "shared laughter."

Evaluative reactions

Finally, some listeners' responses were placed in a third category, that of evaluative responses to the therapist. The responses however were not made concerning each therapist. It was therefore not possible to present the data as with the previous categories. The responses were both positive and negative. "Good response" was one of the positive reactions. "I had a warm feeling," was another.

Yet, therapists were accused by two of the listeners as using too many "yes, uh-huhs," and "putting a stamp of approval on bitching." One therapist was charged with "talking too much" and of being "too intense." One listener noted that the therapist talked so much that it was the client who was saying, "yes, uh-huh."

A listener wondered whether the therapists were really listening and understanding the significance their clients' feelings and experiences. Another listener believed that some therapist responses seemed to interrupt the flow of the clients' thought and experience. He observed that on some occasions "when the therapists responded, the clients would often stop to confirm the response." In addition, a listener noted that there were several times that therapists talked at the same time as the client.

Finally, a listener observed the termination of a session by saying "there was an abrupt ending of the session."

Therapists' observations

The first item in the therapists' questionnaire was: Indicate how you characteristically practice person-centered therapy. All six therapists made reference to Rogers or the practice of his theory. "My practice fits the description in the writings of Carl R. Rogers," wrote one therapist. Another wrote, "I live the spirit of the core conditions." A third wrote, "I embody values-attitudes of CCT." And, "I related primarily through empathic understanding response process." Another stated, "I define my major conscious attempt and intent and the only goal to be empathic with the client; i.e., to understand from their perspective what their world is like." Still another stated, "I listen carefully, check my understanding of the client's experience with the client and encourage them to reflect on their experience." And the last wrote, "I focus on the client's unfolding awareness —reflect, clarify and also use dome gestalt/existential theory to ground experimental work."

A second item was: Characterize the person who seems to benefit from your approach. One therapist stated, "Different kinds of people: 15 to 50, religious, agnostic, atheist, in great psychic pain who had major difficulties in terms of their emotional needs met in childhood." Another response was, "People who have not been helped to develop a workable philosophy of life." Others who seem to benefit from PCA are persons who "have not had an adequate role model," or "people who have been typically out of touch with their inner selves." Another therapist stated that one likely to benefit from the approach is the "person experiencing at least a vague incongruence…feeling some anxiety." "The person…needs to be motivated toward therapy," wrote one therapist. And another said a person seem to benefit from the approach when he or she "perceives to some minimal degree the realness, caring and understanding of my self." One response stated that "all types of people, types of problems, types of illnesses, etc." benefit from the therapists approach. Another therapist wrote, "Characteristics are irrelevant if I can accomplish the empathic stance." Another wrote, "A few have not wanted to work with me. They have expressed a desire for more control from the therapist or of being interested in psychoanalytic type interpretation."

One therapist responded by making a statement about a person who would not be helped. He or she would be "someone on drugs, or drunk, someone completely self absorbed, someone absolutely self absorbed, someone absolutely defensive." Another statement in this fashion was, "I have least success with substance abuse in the denial phase. (These folks need more 'tough love' than I am comfortable with.)."

The third item was: In regards to the therapeutic session you are sending to us, what do you believe are the key experiences for you? It was interesting to note that some responses were centered on the client's key experiences rather than the therapist's experiences. One therapist wrote a key experience was related to the "client reporting insight." Another response described key experiences as when the "client shifted from focusing on annoyance…to empathic concern." Another key experience for a therapist was when the "client expressed sensitive awareness…that her attitudes and/or behavior may have contributed to her husband feeling embarrassed." Still another response stated that a key experience occurred in the "client's recognition that, just as she was able to help herself, the sister-in-law has the capacity to help herself make constructive changes."

One therapist did share responses concerning key experiences for himself. He stated that he "said very little." He wrote, "I spoke to clarify my understanding of what the person meant." Another therapist said a key experience for him was when "we both ended the session laughing." One therapist seemed offended by the question: "I do not believe there are necessarily (nor even usually) key moments in helping relations.… I think it is a mistake to think in these terms about therapy. Why are you?"

Clients' Observations

The first item on the clients' questionnaire asked for the characteristics of the therapeutic relationship which the client found helpful or significant.

The responses were simple. Clients responded to the question by describing therapists as having "warmth," "honesty," "empathy," "freedom," "humor," "acceptance," "sincerity," "reliability," "dependability," and "trust."

Therapists were described as being "caring," "loving," "dependable," "open," "without judgment," "supportive," "genuine," "honest" and "giving." One client stated that his therapist was "not a textbook therapist." Another noted that a helpful characteristic for him was that his therapist smiled at him during therapy.

Other characteristics of the therapist included: "laughs," has "similar ideas to mine," is "not bound by solidified image," "listens," "human," "understands," that "he liked me," the therapist "listened," and "agreed with me that love feels good."

The second item asked of the clients was: in regards to this present session, what do you regard as being key experiences for you? One client stated, "Moving toward a greater congruence between self and ideal, awareness of experiences previously not realized, identifying inconsistencies in thought processes, changing value system and experience close relationship with the therapist." Another's key experiences included, "Sensing of feeling of progress of hope. Feeling a sense of panic over age. Indecision about marriage—feeling trapped. And hopeful to resolve innate confusion."

Another client's key experiences involved "separating two contradictory, conflicting parts." The client also stated, "I learned by looking and interacting with each part of me."

Still another client wrote, "I was able to understand better. I felt like a subject instead of a victim."

Finally, one client said that a key experience was "a sense of being understood." "I can find my way," the client wrote.

Conclusions

Listeners' Perspective

Remarks from listeners who participated in this study seemed to fit three general categories concerning the characteristics of person-centered relationships. The first characteristic of the person-centered therapeutic relationship is that person-centered therapists have observable personal characteristics. In this study the traditional Rogerian characteristics (1957, 1961, 1980) of empathy, positive regard (acceptance, warmth) and congruence (genuineness) were noted. However, a number of other characteristics were noted including "inviting," "patient," "enthusiastic," "agreeable," "easygoing," "relaxed," "tender," "not surprised," "receptive," "dominating," "gentle," "soft," "spontaneous," "interested," "concerned," "accepting," "friendly," having a "sense of humor." "comfortable," "silent," "sensitive," "soothing," "curious," "responsive" "open," "kind." "reactive." "permitting," and "sharing."

A second characteristic is that "techniques" or "styles" of the therapists can be noted. While these "techniques" were not formal, such as recognized by such schools of therapy as psychoanalysis (i.e. dream interpretation, or free association) or Behaviorism (relaxation, or desensitization), certain characteristics were regarded as techniques when the investigator reviewed the listeners' data.

The first technique was the common use of "yes, uh-huh." Other observations seen as techniques included, "nonconfrontive," "attempted to understand," "focused on feelings," "reflective," "summarizing," "interruptive," "interpretive." "clarifies," "explores," "attentive," "confrontive," "active," "speculative," "silence," "encouraging," "asks questions," "laughs," "made comparisons," "self-disclosure," and "shared observations."

The third characteristic is that the relationship fostered evaluative responses in observers who participated in the study. These responses were positive and negative. "Good response" was one of the positive reactions. "I had a warm feeling" was another.

There were also negative reactions. Therapists were accused of using too many "yes, uh-huhs," "putting a stamp of approval on bitching," "talking too much," were too "interruptive" and of being "too intense." One listener wondered whether or not the therapists were really listening and understanding the significance of the feelings and experiences of the clients. Another listener stated that the therapist "puts words into the client's mouth."

It was noted that clients stopped what they were saying to respond to therapists. Thus, the therapists seemed to interrupt the client.

Therapists' Perspectives

Data from the therapists presented other characteristics of the person-centered therapeutic relationship. The first item, "indicate how you characteristically practice person-centered therapy," demonstrated that six therapists felt that they adhered to Rogers' theory. All the therapists claimed to have been strongly influenced by Rogers and to adhere to the attitudinal qualities of unconditional positive regard, empathy and congruence.

The second item, "characterize the person who seems to benefit from your approach," indicates that the therapists who participated in this study, as a group, believe that virtually anyone can benefit from person-centered therapy. The therapists indicated that they provide therapy for a wide range of persons and problems. As long as therapists feel they can maintain the core conditions, the potential for therapy is there for all kinds of people.

The lone reservations concerning this issue pertain to those clients who wish to have a more directive style of therapy and those who are intoxicated by drugs or alcohol. It was indicated that persons could not benefit from this approach if they did not want to be assisted by nondirective means or were too defensive.

Responses to the third item, "in regards to the therapeutic session you are sending to us, what do you believe are the key experiences for you," indicated that in the person-centered therapeutic relationship a therapist might define key experiences in terms of the client's key experiences. Another therapist might indeed notice key experiences for himself or herself. Yet another therapist might not believe there are such things as key experiences.

Clients' Perspectives

Characteristics of the therapeutic relationship can also be derived from the data of the clients. The first item asking for the characteristics of the therapeutic relationship which the client found helpful or significant facilitated a wide range of characteristics including, "warmth," "honesty," "empathy," "freedom," "humor," "acceptance," "sincerity," "reliability," "dependability," "trust," "caring," "loving," "dependable," "open," "without judgment," "supportive," "genuine," "honest," and "giving" to represent a few.

The second item, "what do you regard as being key experiences for you?" indicated that clients in the person-centered therapeutic relationship do have key experiences. No client denied having key experiences or even failed to answer the question concerning key experiences.

It was noted that clients had no negative comments. There were no complaints. No statements of disappointment were noted. In fact, several clients stated that they had been in therapy with other therapists and that their present therapist had been the most helpful.

Issues of Interest

The first issue of interest involves the observation that the therapist disappeared. One observer noted that the "client might as well have been talking to a brick wall." Another stated, "I cannot tell if the therapist makes a difference here." one of the investigators who also served as one of the listeners noted that he "lost track of the therapist." one listener simply said that one therapist "disappeared."

The investigators felt there were two main reasons for this "disappearance." First, if one of the tasks of the therapist is to be empathic and if the therapist accomplishes that task, he or she will enter into the world of the client as if he or she were the client. Thus the focus will be upon the client and the therapist will not be noticed. The investigator also felt that since the primary focus of the therapists were upon the clients, with a secondary focus upon the therapist, observers would periodically loose track of the therapists.

This is interesting in that the study was focused upon discovering something of the therapist, not the client. What was discovered then was that the therapists remained focused on the client and thus got out of the way. Attention was upon the clients in spite of the studies effort to study the therapists.

Still, a second issue concerns the interruption of clients by therapists making responses. observers noted that there were interruptions of the client to make reflective statements. Clients were put in the position of reacting to or verifying the therapists' responses. They thus were side-tracked and interrupted in order to keep the therapists on track. It was noted that one client was interrupted so much by a therapist who appeared to be on target with his statements that she was reduced to saying "Uh-huh," and listening.

It was noted, however, that none of the clients made any complaints about these interruptions. They reported having key experiences and seemed to the investigator to move on with their issues in spite of the interruptions.

A third issue is the question of issue of who benefits from person-centered therapy. Some therapists felt that they could not define any particular characteristics of persons who could not be helped by the client-centered/person-centered therapy. It was felt that virtually any person, young or old, religious or nonreligious with any kind of problem could be helped.

Therapists did indicate that there were people who could not benefit, those who were intoxicated, or who wanted a different style of therapy.

Inferences

The Therapeutic Relationship

Rogers' definition of therapy is the reorganization of the self (Rogers, 1951, 1961, 1980). The therapeutic relationship then would be a specific relationship in which an environment is created for the alteration of the self to take place. This study revealed many characteristics of that relationship. Since only six therapists were studies, it suggests other characteristics would be present, though it does not suggest that any particular characteristics are therapeutic.

In this study, the person-centered therapeutic relationship is one in which the personal characteristics of the therapist can be noted, techniques or styles can be noted, and key experiences emerge for therapists and clients.

Many types of persons who can benefit from the client-centered/person-centered therapy with the limits being in regards to clients who wish to have a more directive approach, or who are intoxicated.

The attitudinal qualities of empathy, unconditional regard and congruence were noted. Yet many other characteristics were noted. These characteristics, while not being empathic or unconditional regard states, were regarded as being genuine and idiosyncratic by the investigator. Thus, the attitudinal quality of congruence may be seen as containing many other characteristics of person-centered therapists.

Since the therapeutic relationship comprises a wide variety of characteristics and since there are differences between therapists, it can be inferred that each therapist is idiosyncratic as a person, and perhaps even differing during other therapeutic sessions (a research project similar to this one could study could a series of sessions).

Summary

This was a qualitative investigation which sought to discover anew characteristics of selected person-centered therapeutic relationships. It was discovered that in these relationships characteristics of the person-centered therapist emerge, that there is a use of technique (though not like those of other therapeutic approaches), that the sessions can evoke evaluative responses on the part of observers, that there are key experiences for the therapists and the clients, and that therapists believe their approach can be of benefit to a wide range of persons.

While the attitudinal qualities of empathy, unconditional positive regard and congruence were noted, it was also noted that a wide range of idiosyncratic therapist and relationship characteristic emerged as well.

Three issues of interest were noted. First, the issue of the "disappearance" of the therapist which the investigator felt was due in part to the condition of empathy. Second, clients were often interrupted and had to stop the directions they had chosen in order to address the responses or comments of the therapists. And last, it was felt that there were no particular sorts of persons who could not be helped by person-centered therapy except those who wished to have a more directive style of therapy or those who under the influence of drugs or alcohol.

References

Bower, D. W. (1985). Assumptions and attitudes of the Rogerian person-centered approach to counseling: Implications for pastoral counseling. Unpublished research project, Columbia Theological Seminary, Atlanta, Ga.

Bower, D. W. (1989). The attributes of five person-centered therapists. Unpublished doctoral dissertation, University of Georgia, Athens, Ga.

Glaser, B. G., & Strauss, A, L. (1967). **The discovery of grounded theory: strategies for qualitative research**. New York: Aldine de Gruyter.

Goetz, J. P., & LeCompte, M. D. (1984). **Ethnography and qualitative design in educational research**. Orlando: Academic Press.

Patton, M. Q. (1980). **Qualitative evaluation methods**. Beverly Hills: Sage.

Rogers, C. R. (1957). The necessary and sufficient conditions of therapeutic change. Journal of Consulting Psychology, 21, 95-103.

Rogers, C. R. (1951). **Client-centered therapy**. Boston: Houghton Mifflin.

Rogers, C. R. (1961). **On becoming a person**. Boston: Houghton Mifflin.

Rogers, C. R. (1980). **A way of being**. Boston: Houghton Mifflin.

Strauss, A. L. (1987). **Qualitative analysis of social scientists**. Cambridge: Cambridge University Press.

Strauss, A. L., & Corbin, J. (1990). **Basic qualitative research**. London: Sage.

Applications

Application of the Person-Centered Approach in Daily Life

Jody DeRidder

Those of us in America today live in a society marked by alienation and loneliness. As the population has grown, our life has been increasingly defined by our submersion in the masses. The majority of communication directed toward us does not recognize us as individuals, nor does it invite feedback: for the communicators behind television and advertisements, newspapers, magazines, mass mailings and company memos, we have become part of the unknown crowd, interesting only insofar as we can be manipulated. Bureaucracies and mechanized industrial labor have developed to meet the needs of the majority, at the cost of the individual (Bryant, 1971; Gerson, 1971). As an increasingly mobile workforce has evolved (Forbes, 1979; Pilisuk & Parks, 1986) to meet the demands of the business world, extended families and small, close-knit communities have become nearly obsolete. We no longer have the sense of safety, acceptance, and belonging that were so much a part of our forebearers' world. As small towns have become cities, suburbs have replaced communities. Rarely do neighbors even have contact with one another anymore, beyond the perfunctory greeting (Shaffer & Anundsen, 1993). In our crowded cities, privacy is maintained by the avoidance of eye contact. As we avoid contact, we avoid connection; our increasing isolation within the crowd increases stress and fails to feed our hungry souls. The lack of meaningful relationship with others results in a loss of identity, as the alienated person loses touch not only with other persons but also with himself (Gerson). "To a degree probably unknown before, modern man *experiences* his loneliness, his cut-off-ness, his isolation both from his own deeper being and from others" (Rogers, 1989, p. 158).

The extent of impact of this alienation on our current social problems can only be estimated. David Torbett, director of the Family Enrichment foundation in Denver, CO, states, "A significant stress that is both external and internal in its effects and causes comes from living and working in a mechanistic society where emphasis is placed on production and achievement to the exclusion of any kind of human feeling...A direct result of this is the increased incidence of alcoholism, drug addiction, suicides and other stress-related illnesses" (Forbes, 1979, p. 81). Suicide (Teele, 1970) and depression (Brown & Andrews, 1986) are clearly related to stable and durable social relationships. "Progressive social disorganization and disorientation generated by the lack of feedback and the feeling of alienation and hopelessness may also lead to various types of psychosomatic disturbances even in individuals who may not exhibit gross behavioural pathology" (Corson, 1971, p. 186). Lack of social support coupled with interpersonal stresses has been suggested as a cause of circulatory collapse and death (Lynch, 1977). Feelings of connectedness to other human beings certainly appears to be critical to human health (Pilisuk & Parks, 1986; Selye, 1978). Yet more than fifty million people, 26 percent of Americans, have said that they recently felt lonely (Pilisuk & Parks).

As opportunities for support outside the home have dwindled, pressure to meet interpersonal needs has increased within the nuclear family and dyadic relationships. Romance is stressed in popular culture as a solution to all our needs, symbolic of complete and total acceptance. Soaring divorce rates testify to the inability of marriage to meet current needs and expectations. "It is in the marital role that husband and wife seek support and solace in the face of stress...yet the marital role...has itself become a stressful role" (Palmer, 1981, p. 163). A major cause of this stress between couples is due to a dissimilarity of expectations (Torbutt, 1979). It seems that if we could learn how to more clearly *communicate* our needs and expectations with one another, and could *hear* another's viewpoints with compassion and empathy, we could open the dialogue to create hope and change in even these stressful situations (Rogers, 1980).

Few of us recognize that we have the resources to address these concerns. By and large, we throw up our hands in helpless frustration, unable to imagine how to create change. Increasingly, people of all ages are escaping from the pressures of their lives into the voyeuristic and displaced emotional release of television drama (Kabat-Zinn, 1990). The drawback to this is that when we turn off the tube, our problems remain.

Watching television often prevents you from engaging in meaningful conversations with others about the problems and successes of the day. This verbal communication can be an effective tool in releasing tension. Avoidance of communication by substituting television watching can actually be masking serious problems which need to be worked out to preserve a healthy parent-child relationship or even a faltering marriage (Forbes, 1979, p.22). Continued avoidance is not a solution. While dependence on helping personnel such as counselors, psychologists, and other professional helping groups is growing, it cannot replace the emotional support that once came from extended families, friends, and neighbors (Lynch, 1977); nor can everyone afford to pay for such a necessity. The healing of America's loneliness will not happen en masse at the hands of counselors, but as a result of a grassroots movement towards connection and caring.

Those who offer hope in the face of this morbid state of affairs focus on small group origins of interpersonal caring, a self-help movement to reweave the interpersonal fabric of our lives and communities, and the need for us not only to come together as individuals, but also to connect into circles connected to other such circles around the globe (Pilisuk & Parks, 1986). As a method for learning to connect, the person-centered approach offers a ray of hope, a tool for change. It offers possibilities for personal growth and development, and demands practice and compassion to integrate it into our lives. Trying something new requires courage, especially when it touches on our own sense of identity: who we are, and how we are.

The person-centered approach is, as Carl Rogers termed it, "a way of being". An eminent psychologist, he developed the approach first for use in therapy and counseling, and later expanded the application to education, business, groups, communities, and even politics (Rogers, 1980; Rogers, 1989). The three central tenants are: congruence (being real, or genuine), unconditional positive regard (acceptance, caring, prizing the other), and empathy (sensing the feelings and personal meanings the other is experiencing—and communicating this to the other person) (Rogers, 1980). Using this approach in our everyday interactions offers us the possibility of new richness and depth of interconnection with others. So much of our current interaction is colored by our presuppositions about people: what we have decided about them, based on our past experiences. We are quick to judge, and no longer take the time or the opportunity to really *listen*, with an open mind. If we are willing to make this one change, a whole new world will open to us, for we will discover that people aren't who we thought they were (Rogers, 1980)…and neither are we. In opening the avenues to rich, real communication, we are opening the door to discovery, to growth, to healing…to the possibilities of discovering new perspectives and hope.

When we listen to the other, in the person-centered approach, we are trying to understand the topic *through that person's eyes* (Rogers, 1961). We honor his or her right to whatever point of view they have, and respect it as we would want our own point of view respected. We learn to disagree with respect, accepting our differences: honoring one another as worthwhile people, regardless. Being congruent, being real, we do not hide our feelings and thoughts, but we take *responsibility* for them (Rosenberg, 1983; Shaffer & Anundsen, 1993). The other is not to blame for our feelings; the other person is just as worthy as we ourselves are. There *is* no "Us vs. Them"; we're all in this together. Slowly, interaction after interaction, the world becomes all "us", for we begin to see each of "them" as real individuals, worthy of our compassion and respect.

Embracing the person-centered approach requires a willingness to change, to open to possibilities that may require us to readjust our patterns of thinking and behaving, even our attitudes, however long-standing. A willingness to truly hear the other, even when we disagree, implies non-defensiveness, an acceptance of responsibility for one's emotions and preferences, and a willingness to not impose those preferences on the world around us. Relinquishing the effort to control others and events in order to make them more acceptable to ourselves, is a difficult but necessary task. Accepting that one's own viewpoint is not the only valid one is often frightening, for it implies that no one has the corner on the truth; there *is* no "solid rock" on which to stand.

It appears to me that the way of the future must be to base our lives and our education on the assumption that there are as many realities as there are persons, and that our highest priority is to accept that hypothesis and proceed from there. Proceed where? Proceed, each of us, to explore open-mindedly the many, many perceptions of reality that exist. We would, I believe, enrich our own lives in the process. We would also become more able to cope with the reality in which each one of us exists, because we would be aware of many more options. This might well be a life full of perplexity and difficult choices, demanding greater maturity, but it would be an exciting and adventurous life.... Suppose that instead of shutting out the realities of others as absurd or dangerous or heretical or stupid, I was willing to explore and learn about those realities?

Suppose you were willing to do the same. What would be the social result? I think that our society would be based not on a blind commitment to a cause or creed or view of reality, but on a common commitment to each other as rightfully separate persons, with separate realities. The natural human tendency to care for another would no longer be "I care for you because you are the same as I" but, instead, "I prize and treasure you because you are different from me (Rogers, 1980, pp. 104-5).

So adopting the person-centered approach brings us slowly to the task of learning to sit with the "not knowing", the place of being willing to hear all sides and honor their seemingly conflicting validity. Having our own preferred version of the truth becomes recognized as just that: not as the *objective* truth, but as one of many *subjective* truths.

This stance allows us to honor others as equals, with respect for and willingness to consider differing and sometimes difficult points of view. (I consider this "unconditional positive regard", as the prerequisite is to suspend judgement and be willing to view the other person's viewpoint as valid.) This stance allows for empathy, as we enter into the world of another person, seeking to see and experience the world through his or her eyes. This stance allows for congruence, being real and true to ourselves, for we are *not* required to abandon our personal preferences, our personal truths. On the contrary, it is incumbent upon us to share with others our own experiences, our own truths, that they may then come to know us as well. And in this sharing, true connection is born.

Applications in the Home

Possibly the most difficult place for us to apply the person-centered approach is with those nearest and dearest to us, as these relationships may already have become so structured that any change may be perceived as threatening. And yet, these are the most important relationships we have; if we do not seek true connection here, with an attitude of caring and willingness to honor and respect differences, than we have truly abandoned a precious possibility. People can be married for many years and never truly come to know one another due to the felt necessity to play formal roles in that relationship (Jourard, 1964). The answer is to open the relationship up to the possibilities of congruent disclosure and willingness to empathize and prize one another as individuals. A healthy relationship is defined by the willingness to share, and be shared with; by the valuing of one another; by the sharing of power; and by the honoring of differences (Wotitz, 1993).

Habitual stances in the face of what we dislike from one another is the most critical place to bring the person-centered approach. And the first element of change is this: to recognize that our emotional reaction stems from our preferences, rather than from the other's behavior (Rosenberg, 1977).

For example, imagine that your spouse has just made a large purchase without consulting you beforehand. You may be feeling several things: frightened over how to now pay pending bills; angry that you weren't consulted, and hurt that your concerns weren't considered. In this situation, your preferences (that were not met) would perhaps be: 1) that necessary expenses be met before any other purchases are made; 2) that you talk together about large expenditures prior to purchase; and 3) that your concerns be considered and honored when decisions are made that affect you both. If you did *not* have these preferences, you would not be feeling frightened, angry and hurt; you might be a little puzzled, if this was unusual behavior, or you might not even notice. Obviously, having these preferences (or others like them) is what underlies the existence of the pain, anger, and fear. Recognizing this allows you to take responsibility for your feelings, for you chose these preferences. No one chose them for you! The other's actions did not create your feelings, and your spouse may have very different preferences and concerns. Until you can hear each other's viewpoints with empathy and respect, you will not be able to resolve the issue in a manner that will heal the breach that has occurred between you. Miscommunication, lack of communication, and misunderstandings are the basis of much of our suffering in relationship. The use of empathy, congruence, and unconditional positive regard offers the basis for healing the damage caused, and creating a new path toward deeper, more healthy relating (Rogers, 1961).

Once you take responsibility for your feelings, and recognize that your spouse may have a point of view you may have not yet fully understood, you can begin to approach the problem. Stating your feelings is a good place to start! Your spouse may be totally surprised and disturbed by your reaction——and willing to hear what preferences led to your emotions. If however, his/her reaction is defensive, openly stating that you value him/her regardless of what has happened, and showing an interest in hearing what led to the purchase, is perhaps a better place to start. This would be using unconditional positive regard and empathy to explore the situation. Listening with a willingness to truly understand may help to dissipate your anger and hurt, as you begin to see another perspective on the situation. Then it is important to share your own feelings, and the preferences that underlie them, taking full responsibility for them so the other does not feel blamed or judged negatively. If both partners can come to feel truly heard, without the experience of attack, new lines of communication and sharing will be forged. Perceived attack triggers defensiveness; defensiveness creates barriers to hearing and caring; communication is hampered (if not completely stalled). Non-defensive open disclosure and empathy create the possibility of deeply enhanced communication. As each feels their perspectives honored and respected, as each feels fully heard and cared for, the path for healing and growth begins to open.

Applications in the Workplace

Many of the work environments in the US are deeply bureaucratic and autocratic. Employees are not valued as people, with feelings, need, desires and concerns; they are often treated as objects, extensions of the machines with which they work (Zork, 1993). This depersonalized environment is dehumanizing and disempowering. The attitudes inherent in these systems undermine employees' sense of self worth, and create barriers to communication, change, and growth (Gardell, 1971). Employees are rarely recognized and respected for the valuable human resources they have to offer, but instead are viewed as liabilities, cost overhead, and barriers to "progress" (McGregor, 1960). The question that arises here is, to what are we progressing?

The transformation in economics must start with a renewal of human values, and a growing need to reassert them in the way we value activity and productivity. Our infatuation with mechanisms has led us to elevate the automatic, machine-like functioning of the market to be the highest value in economics. We treat the market as if it is able to make moral decisions. As a result, society has become increasingly insensitive and lacking in compassion (Tibbs, 1998, p. 27). If the bottom line is more important than the damage done to the Earth and our fellow inhabitants, where is the value in that? What accomplishment is so worthy that the ends outweigh the means? Incredible wealth may be amassed, but if the wake of destruction is deep and wide, where is the profit? "Money-world institutions are human creations. We have both the right and the power to change them when they no longer serve our needs" (Korten, 1996, p. 21).

The first two requirements for any company to qualify for *The 100 Best Companies to Work for in America* are: "1. Make people feel that they are part of a team or, in some cases, a family...2. Encourage open communication, informing...people of new developments and encouraging them to offer suggestions and complaints" (Levering & Moskowitz, 1984, p. ix). This is a basic recognition of the human need for connection and communication. Worker satisfaction has been correlated with the opportunity for increased interactions with others on the job (Gross, 1970). There is always the argument that we do not have enough time to interact with one another. If we do not make the time to be there for each other, we are choosing to lose the possibility to create a more humane and healthy future—-both for ourselves and for our children. The benefits to be gained by respecting, honoring, and validating those we see in daily life run much deeper than our wallets. To build a network of caring individuals to whom one can relate, with whom one can feel heard, is life-affirming, and creates the basis for hope and change. We will all die, and in the end what matters most is how we've touched each other's lives. Therefore, any human compassion we can bring to the workplace will be more than worth the effort, in human terms. When people become cogs in the great machine, we have lost our hope.

The alternative is to recognize each other as brothers and sisters, struggling to do our best in difficult situations; and to honor what each has to offer. By bringing unconditional positive regard into the workplace, we bring respect, and a starting ground for connection. And upon that ground, we need to plant empathy and congruence.

Congruence is another seriously missing element of hope in the workplace. The workplace is filled with unspoken rules to fulfill an image instead of speak the truth. Unspoken rules dominate, such as "appear in control, appear to have all the answers, don't show weakness". From the initial interview, where we seek to show only the qualities that will get us what we want (the job), we learn to keep our truths to ourselves, and control every impression we give to the people around us. Careers and fortunes are balanced on impression manipulation: how well can we convince the other to give us what we want? Not only does this reduce the other person to an object to be manipulated, it reduces us to the same thing, by default (Rogers, 1989a). We expect to be used by our employer for as long as we appear to be worth the cost, and then cast aside: "downsized". There is no room in this equation for human faults and feelings and needs, no room for compassion and honest sharing, no room for the birth of creativity. Our markets suffer from this, as other cultures far surpass our products and research development. Where it is not safe to fail, it is not safe to risk...where it is not safe to risk, new ideas will not be ventured (Rogers, 1961).

There is also the human cost. We put on our mask as we go out the door in our work clothes, our costume/uniform. We set our selves aside, or try to, in order to meet the harsh demands of our work. But to what extent do we really succeed? How long can we fool ourselves that how we really feel doesn't affect our work? And what price do we pay for submerging our true selves in allegiance to the company, in trade for our paychecks? High blood pressure, heart attacks, ulcers, substance and alcohol abuse, spouse and child abuse, obesity and innumerable other symptoms point to a culture stressed to the breaking point. Is this how we want to live? Is this how we want our children to live? Our society's work atmosphere is one of domination, control, competition, power politics and game-playing. There is a serious lack of truth and integrity present in almost every interaction, for fear of "losing face", power, or perceived control of a situation (and therefore, its outcome). However, some companies are moving in the direction of shared power (Dominguez, 1998; Uehling, 1997). Some wonderful research on the effects of collaborative power has been done by Peggy Natiello:

Relationships that develop in a climate of collaborative power are characterized by certain qualities: (1) openness (all information is fully shared), (2) responsiveness (all needs and ideas are carefully heard), (3) dignity (everyone is respected and considered), (4) personal empowerment (each person affected feels free and responsible to participate fully), (5) alternating influence (impact on group process moves from one person to another as a result of self-awareness, wisdom, experience, or expressed need), and (6) cooperation rather than competition. (1990, p. 272)

And yet the perceived risk of being real, of claiming our integrity, seems valid. It is possible that contracts will be lost, jobs may be lost, allies may be lost, with the revelation of vulnerability and honest feeling (Shaffer & Anundsen, 1993). And what will be there to take the place of these things? True connection, hopefully. We would have to seek out and create work environments that encourage honesty and openness instead of games and politics. We would begin to create a work culture that values people as individuals, as true human resources, with possibilities far beyond any job title.

Then again, taking the risk of being congruent in our present workplace may have the opposite effect of what we fear. The change may be so surprising and refreshing, that our co-workers, supervisors, employees, clients and "competitors" may be taken aback for a moment, only to find they truly appreciate knowing exactly where they stand with us. "Cutting to the chase" has a power all its own. It breaks through the manipulations, the confusions, the deceptions and endless machinations that fill our work hours and add to our stress levels, without improving our products or our lives.

There are no easy answers. A wise person has said that the greatest journey begins with a single step...and our challenge is to face our fears and take that step. And then another. And another. And before long we may find we have company on our path, and that the rewards of the path chosen are well worth the cost. Our humanity hangs in the balance, and our hope for fulfillment as human beings. Will we sell our souls to the system that daily spews out remnants of once-idealistic brothers and sisters? How long can we deceive ourselves that we will be different, that we will not pay the price for suppressing our spirits, our feelings, our needs and ideas, our hopes and dreams? It is a sad delusion that keeps us beating our heads on the brick walls of this prison we have constructed. Better to take the prison down, one brick at a time...one truth at a time. This way lies hope. It will take a grassroots effort to create change in our dehumanizing workplace environments, but it can be done. Step by step—one person at a time. As we begin the movement, it will grow, like a wave, as others sigh in relief to see it can be done, that the fears can be faced, that people can be real with each other in the workplace and the world does not end.

What have we to lose? We have already lost ourselves. It is time to reclaim our humanity and our integrity.

Applications in the Community

A major complaint in both cities and suburbs today is that there is no sense of community (Shaffer & Anundsen, 1993). Neighbors are transient, as success in the workplace arena often demands travel and relocation. Many are unwilling to expend the time and energy to "put down roots", knowing the time will soon come when they will likely move on. We as a culture seem to be afraid to risk involvement for fear of loss and pain when it ends or changes. So we increase our sense of alienation and isolation, often blaming the other for not being friendly, or blaming outside forces beyond our control, rather than taking responsibility for helping to create our own isolation. In the process we lose something precious: *connection*. Contact. The fertilizer that enhances our growth and well-being, that offers us opportunity for change and new perspectives, that offers us support and personal challenge. Jourard has said that "no man can come to know himself except as an outcome of disclosing himself to another person.... [Disclosure is] the index of man functioning at his highest and truly human level rather than at the level of a thing or an animal. Self-disclosure, however, requires courage. Not solely the courage to be...but the courage to be known" (1964, pp. 6-7).

There is no solution for fear besides courage. As long as we allow fear to rule us, we are trapped and crippled by it, unable to create change and growth. As we face our fears and begin to walk through them, they fall away, and a whole new perspective is gained, along with a sense of strength. Realization dawns that *it is within our power* to create change and improve our lives.

But the first step is always the hardest. Taking advantage of the few opportunities we have to connect with one another is difficult, but a necessary beginning place. When is the last time you asked the check-out clerk at the grocery store about his or her day? When your neighbor was acting strangely, moody or angry, and you ventured over to voice your concern, offering an opportunity for sharing? "Empathy dissolves alienation. For the moment, at least, the recipient finds himself or herself a connected part of the human race" (Rogers, 1980, p. 151). What a gift you have to offer! These and other options lay the beginning foundation for creating connection between our disconnected lives.

A further step would be to *create* more opportunity for intimacy: invite a neighbor over for coffee or dinner, or to join you in an activity; offer to assist someone regularly who could obviously use the help; start a small group in your neighborhood based around a regular potluck or topic of concern. There are many ways to begin relationships (Shaffer & Anundsen, 1993). The mode of meeting will, with attention and care, begin to be less important than the meeting and sharing itself. Reaching out is an expression of congruence on your part, if one truly wants more and deeper connections; and it offers others the opportunity to respond, if they also are ready and willing to move in that direction.

One of the first challenges to establishing new relationships will likely be your own reluctance to value differences. When a neighbor expresses a viewpoint to you which you find disagreeable, how can you respond with empathy and unconditional positive regard, and still maintain your congruence? The key point here is to recognize that just because you disagree does not mean either of you is less worthy as human beings. Each speaks out of current understanding, based on previous experiences——and those understandings and experiences may be very different. Acknowledging these differences and exploring them to gain a greater understanding of one another is the alternative to creating barriers and walls between you. A willingness to explore the experiences that led to those assumptions and beliefs will open the door to real connection and the possibility of growth for both participants. People are not likely to examine their beliefs and the underlying assumptions unless they feel safe and welcomed to do so. This is a gift of empathy and unconditional positive regard: they create a safe and welcoming environment for exploration and growth. Those to whom you offer these qualities will value your presence and be more open to hearing *your* beliefs once they feel fully heard, understood, and valued (Rosenberg, 1977).

Just because you do not agree with the other, there is no need to close the door on them; why should you? Fear? Of what? If we fear to hear the other out, we are afraid that new perspectives will require us to change our own point of view. "It is impossible to be accurately perceptive of another's inner world if you have formed an evaluative opinion of that person" (Rogers, 1980, p. 154). And if we fear to share our point of view, we are acting to prevent rejection rather than creating an opportunity to air our differences and consider one another's arguments and experiences as valid. Closing out those with whom we disagree may give us a sense of righteousness, but it leaves us alone and isolated, connected only with those few with whom we agree. Where is the opportunity for growth in this? Where is the richness of diversity and challenge? Down this path lies only empty loneliness.

Dialogue is necessary to life. "It involves the sharing of thoughts, physical sensations, ideas, ideals, hopes, and feelings. In sum, dialogue involves the reciprocal sharing of any and all life experiences" (Lynch, 1977, p. 217). Without it, we are truly isolated and alone; we have no venue for interpersonal growth and support. For the person who can transform his relationships into true connection, as embodied in "I-Thou" as opposed to "I-It", through true recognition of and honoring of the other as well as of oneself, the world has opened, the light has entered (Buber, 1970). m"No man is an island" is the old saying, yet our society has become such that we often experience ourselves as very much alone and disconnected. Yet we have the opportunity to create change in our lives; in our homes, in our workplace, and in our communities.

If we accept as a basic fact of all human life that we live in separate realities; if we can see those differing realities as the most promising resource for learning in all the history of the world; if we can live together in order to learn from one another without fear; if we can do all this, then a new age could be dawning. (Rogers, 1989a, p. 428)

The person-centered approach gives us the tools to open doors to increased connection and the possibility of growth and healing. In connection lies hope for the future: a more humane and caring future for us all. It is up to us.

Jody DeRidder is presently a graduate student and graduate teaching assistant at the University of Tennessee in Knoxville.

References

Brown, G., & Andrews, B. (1986). Social support and depression. In M. Apple & R. Trumbull (Eds.), **Dynamics of stress: Physiological, psychological, and social perspectives**. New York: Plenum Press.

Bryant, C. (1971). Problems of alienation and disaffection. In C. Bryant (Ed.), **Social problems today: Dilemmas and decencies**. Philadelphia: J.B. Lippincott.

Buyer, M. (1970). **I and thou**. New York: Charles Scribner's Sons.

Corson, S. (1971). The lack of feedback in today's societies—A psychosocial stressor. In L. Levi (Ed.), **Society stress and disease, vol. 1: The psychosocial environment and psychosomatic disease**. London: Oxford University Press.

Dominguez, A. (1998, July 3). Firm dispenses with formal managers. **The Knoxville News Sentinel**, (Associated Press), B1.

Forbes, R. (1979). **Life stress**. Garden City, NY: Doubleday & Co.

Gardell, B. (1971). Alienation and mental health in the modern industrial environment. In L. Levi (Ed.), **Society stress and disease, vol. 1: The psychosocial environment and psychosomatic diseases**. London: Oxford University Press.

Gerson, W. (1971). Alienation in mass society: Some causes and responses. In C. Bryant (Ed.), **Social problems today: Dilemmas and decenciess**. Philadelphia: J.B. Lippincott.

Gross, E. (1970). Work, organization and stress. In S. Levine & N. Scotch (Eds.), **Social stress**. Chicago: Aldine Publishing Co.

Jourard, S. (1964). **The transparent self**. New York: D. Van Nostrand.

Kabat-Zinn, J. (1990). **Full catastrophe living: Using the wisdom of your body and mind to face stress, pain, and illness**. New York: Dell Publishing.

Korten, D. (1996, Fall). Money vs. life. **Yes! A Journal of Positive Futures**, 49-51.

Levering, R., Moskowitz, M., & Katz, M. (1984). **The hundred best companies to work for in America**. Reading, MA: Addison-Wesley Publishing Co.

Lynch, J. (1977). **The broken heart**. New York: Basic Books.

McGregor, D. (1960). **The human side of enterprise**. New York: McGraw-Hill.

Natiello, P. (1990). The person-centered approach, collaborative power, and cultural transformation. **The Person-Centered Review**, 5, 268-86.

Palmer, S. (1981). **Rolestresss: How to handle everyday tension**. Englewood Cliffs, NJ: Prentice Hall.

Pilisuk, M., & Parks, S. (1986). **The healing web: Social networks and human survival**. Hanover, NH: University Press of New England.

Rogers, C. R. (1961). **On becoming a person**. Boston: Houghton Mifflin Co.

Rogers, C. R. (1980). **A way of being**. Boston: Houghton Mifflin Co.

Rogers, C. R. (1989a). **Carl Rogers Dialogues**. H. Kirschenbaum & V. Henderson (Eds.) Boston: Houghton Mifflin Co.

Rogers, C. R. (1989b). Ellen West—And loneliness. In H. Kirschenbaum & V. Henderson (Eds.), **The Carl Rogers Reader**. Boston: Houghton Mifflin Co.

Rosenberg, M. (1977). Training materials for nonviolent communication. Sherman, TX: The Center for Nonviolent Communication

Rosenberg, M. (1983). **A model for nonviolent communication**. Sherman, TX: The Center for Nonviolent Communication.

Selye, H. (1978). **The stress of life**. New York: McGraw-Hill, Inc.

Shaffer, C. & Anundsen, K. (1993). **Creating community anywhere: Finding support and connection in a world**. New York: Putnam Publishing Group.

Teele, J. (1970). Social pathology and stress. In S. Levine & N. Scotch (Eds.), **Social stress**. Chicago: Aldine Publishing Co.

Tibbs, H. (1998, Spring). Millenium scenarios. **Yes! A Journal of Positive Futures**, 24-28.

Uehling, M. (1997, Winter). Democracy at work. **Yes! A Journal of Positive Futures**, 40-41.

Wotitz, J. (1993). **The intimacy struggle**. Deerfield Beach, FL: Health Communications, Inc.

Zorc, A. (1993, Summer/Fall). America's top 100 workplaces. **Coop America Quarterly: A Magazine for Building Economic Alternatives**, 16-17.

Person-Centered Mentoring

Doug Bower

The purpose of this chapter is to reflect upon the application of the Person-Centered Approach to mentoring school children. The basic stance of the approach is presented, and the principles of the approach as understood by the author is reviewed in relationship to his experiences as a mentor in the Oglethorpe County School system.

Basic Stance

The basic assumption here of the author is that the Person-Centered Approach maintains: 1) that if an environment rich in the core conditions of empathy, acceptance, and congruence is offered, individuals strive toward being fully themselves, and 2) the individual develops inner and external resources for enhancing and developing the self. We are not born into a vacuum and do not grow alone. Rather we are interdependent on resources within and without to reach our fullest potentials. The "core conditions" represent the external forces needed for personal growth, while self actualization represents the internal forces needed for personal growth.

The attitudes of the core conditions (Bower, 1994) impact the function of the mentor's purpose and participation in the mentoring experience. The purpose becomes one of tending to the experience of the individual who is being mentored. This tending involves the empathic listening process (Brodley, 1982) in balance with the other conditions without carrying expectations as to what will or should be tended to (Bozarth, 1995), or what the outcomes may or may not be. In this, the mentor is not in the role of expert who assumes a position of knowing what is best for the student. The mentor maintains a role as a facilitator for the student who initiates his or her own inherent growth capacities (Rogers, 1959, 1961, 1977). Tending to the experience of the student also means being aware of the factors which contribute to that growth from the immediate world of the student while having limitations of awareness concerning the extent of that world of the student. That is, there is only so much the mentor can learn about the client's experiences. The mentor also is aware of the factors which thwart the emergence of the true self of the student (Bower, 1994).

The mentor's function, then, is related to the maintenance of the attitudinal qualities of empathy, genuineness, and unconditional regard (Bozarth, 1996) in order to create an environment that fosters the emergence of the true self of the student that is (Rogers, 1980). Can this student, as a person, relate to the mentor as a person without many of the limitations society has placed on children relating to adults, or adults relating to children as somehow incapable of functioning fully as the child he or she truly is. Also, can the mentor be open to the experiences of the student who is finding his or her own ways of coping, interacting, and learning in a world that is sometimes misunderstanding, even hostile to those attempts by the student. The idea here is: When a mentoring climate is created, the student is in a position to be in control of his or her life because the actualizing tendency emerges with less encumbrances. The student thus has one more resource for finding ways to become more the person he or she truly is. The student gets more in touch with his or her own creativity and learns to draw of other resources from external sources as well.

Mentoring should not be mistaken for therapy, an environment for the restructuring of the self (Rogers, 1961). However, whenever the core conditions are present the mentoring situation may be therapeutic in that the student is received warmly, respectfully, genuinely, sincerely, and with understanding or at least with attempts to understand. These conditions foster change (Rogers, 1957, 1980).

With the self actualization and formative tendencies as the foundation blocks for of person-centered theory (Bozarth & Brodley, 1986), person-centered mentoring would also be established on that principle. That actualizing tendency is the fulcrum of Roger's theory and is seen as a basic characteristic ingrained in human life with the formative tendency undergirding the whole that is (Bozarth, 1985). These two parallel and complimentary foundation blocks anchor the approach, "Taken together, they are the foundation for the person-centered approach" (Bozarth & Shanks 1989, p. 114). The actualization tendency is the specialized aspect of being human that establishes the uniqueness of being human, mainly the tangible and intangible factors which make it possible for a human being to be a self (Bower, 1985). The formative tendency is a formative process with broader implications in the universe from the formulation of gravity to gather of energy into participles which work together to form planets, stars, and life in general (Rogers, 1961, 1980).

The principles of self-actualization and the formative tendencies can be used as a means of articulating an understanding of students who are mentored using the person-centered approach. The individual student embodies both aspects of these creative processes. The formative tendencies establish the organic mechanisms which make the formulation of the self, the unique self of the individual. Thus, skin, lungs, heart, kidneys, GI tracts, and brain, etc. while not selfs, make it possible for the self to exist. This self is that which evident with thoughts, emotions, and language. Both the body and the self are unique for each individual. Thus perceptions are unique and thus lead to the person-centered approach also being identified as a phenomenological approach. Self actualization specializes in what is uniquely the individual and includes the ability to think, to use a specialized language, weep, cry, and laugh.

Thus the approach offers both an interdependent process which takes factors from the external world while fostering self-organization. There is in this self actualization an ability to put a unique twist to one's own experiences (Jackson, 1981; Lowe 1966; Whitehead, 1978) even though the individual and his or her experiences are similar, but are not the experiences of others. While a number of similarities can be established between human beings, each person is also unique. In a far more complex way, the human being is similar to the snowflake. To our knowledge, no two snowflakes are exactly the same. Each new snowflake offers its own unique twists to what snowflakes look like. So it is with a human being, there are an infinite range of possible twists to what it means to be a human being, and each human being is a complex formulation of those twists.

Yet, we share interdependence, resourcefulness, similar types of physiological structures, and a myriad of experiences which create our unique identities. It is not unusual for a collection of individuals to experience the same emotion together. For instance, when President Kennedy was assassinated, people grieved. Many experienced sadness, many experienced being stunned. It is my opinion that these common experiences or a tendencies to respond to the world in a selective or similar manners, and which sometimes seem to hover at a subconscious level led some theorists like Jung to write about "collective unconscious" (Hall and Lindzey, 1978).

Assumptions

A basic assumption here is that, in the creation of a climate rich in the attitudinal qualities of empathy, genuineness, and unconditional positive regard by a facilitator, a glimpse into the world of the student is more than possible. When this climate is provided an environment promoting personal and interpersonal growth is enhanced not unlike the therapeutic environment of psychotherapy though hardly with the degrees of intensity of therapy, nor with the idea of fostering therapeutic change. As the environment is created, the student will find opportunity for developing self understanding, and become more skilled in developing relationships with others. In this, the student's self-esteem is impacted and confidence is enhanced for present and future interactions. Further, one's ability to make choices becomes improved. The belief here is that the student has the potential and the ability to makes significant self-directed choices which can widen the student's implementation for constructive change related to his or her encounters at school and perhaps at home as well.

I hypothesize that there is a formative directional tendency in the universe, which can be traced and observed in stellar space, in crystals, in microorganisms, in more complex organic life, and in human beings. This is an evolutionary tendency toward greater order, greater complexity, greater interrelatedness. In humankind, this tenency exhibits itself as the individual moves from a single-cell origin to complex organic functioning, to knowing and sensing below the level of consciousness, to a conscious awareness of organism and the external world, to a transcendent awareness of the harmony and unity of the cosmic system, including human kind. (Rogers, 1980, p. 133)

The person-centered environment fosters the student's ability to utilize the actualizing tendency (Rogers, 1969). The student has the freedom to be and become more completely the person he or she truly is as a student in the community of a school when a mentor offers the attitudinal qualities.

These qualities were presented initially by Rogers (1957) as "necessary and sufficient conditions for therapeutic growth." In the 1957, paper Rogers offered six conditions. Later it was found that the conditions were applicable in other disciplines and thus had a wider range of value (Rogers, 1980). The focus over the years, while not discarding the original six conditions, did narrow the field to the "core conditions": genuineness (realness, transparency, or congruence); unconditional positive regard (acceptance, prizing, or caring), and empathy (understanding). The conditions can be described as follows:

Genuineness:

In the mentoring relationship, the mentor is a real person. He or she reveals himself or herself setting aside personal facades (Rogers, 1969, 1980) which would include presuppositions that can utilized by mentors. Facades might also include presuppositions about the student and are not just the psycho-phenomenological fronts. Thus it is important for the mentor to put his or her notions about the student on a shelf (so to speak) so that the mentor can see the student for who he or she is. I handle that in part by asking that teachers and staff not give me their impressions of the student. I often find that when they do give me their observations, I very seldom see the student in the same manner as the person giving me the information. For instance, one student was described to me as a liar. In my experience with the student, I never "caught" him in a lie. In part, my position was one of not expecting him to lie, and not having any authority over him where he had to lie to me. Whether these were actually contributing factors to not being lied to I cannot say, I just never believed I was lied to. Further, even if he had lied to me, it wouldn't have been a problem for me at his age I did some lying myself.

Rogers (1980) described genuineness as being "transparent." The student thus can "see right through what the therapist [mentor] is in the relationship; the client [student] experiences no holding back on the part of the therapist [mentor]" (p. 115). The mentor in this is open to his or own experiences and very much aware of what they are. He or she then reveals those experiences when "appropriate" (Rogers 1980, p. 115). What is the appropriate sharing of the self is determined by the mentor in relationship with the student. There are limitations on this sharing. For instance, the mentor should not scream at the child, using obscenities and put downs. I can of course imagine a mentor having to scream at a child, "Watch out for that falling"

Unconditional positive regard

Bozarth & Shanks (1989) wrote "The therapist experiences a positive, nonjudgmental, accepting attitude toward whatever the client is at the moment." The range of this experience of nonjudgmental is extensive. There is respect of experiences that are not pleasant to encounter. Thus, anger, depression, sadness, have equal value with joy, awe, and celebration. I believe that includes maintaining a positive, nonjudgmental attitude toward the mentor's on range of experiences and that this positive attitude helps the mentor be in charge of his or her experiences. If in charge of his or her experiences, the mentor can prevent adverse feelings from emerging which might be harmful to the student. For instance, it probably is not helpful to feel exasperated with the student and lash out saying, "That was stupid." Such remarks are demoralizing. Further, the mentor who holds his or her own feelings in high regard is likely to hold the feelings and experiences of the students involved.

Rogers (1961, 1969, 1977, 1980) wrote about accepting and prizing persons. This acceptance is unconditional in that the student doesn't have to do anything to earn that acceptance, nor can the student coerce or manipulate the mentor into a position of acceptance or lack of acceptance. Acceptance is not dependent upon the student's behavior.

The danger here with unconditional positive regard seems to me to be the appearance of affirming a variety of heretofore socially unacceptable behavior. For instance, while expressing one's feelings is important, hitting teachers is unacceptable. Grasping the intensity of the situation which led to the adverse behavior is important, but condoning that behavior, even passively, seems inappropriate to me. Does unconditional positive regard foster such negative behavior if the student doesn't have to deal with the consequences of such behavior? That is a tough question to answer, certainly my own concern is that the appearance of condoning disrespectful behavior encourages that behavior. At the same time, perhaps a teacher has violated a student by being disrespectful, coercive and manipulative. If the student doesn't trust that anyone will help, or that the teacher doesn't care, he or she might take matters into his or her own hands and lash out trying protect personal space and integrity.

Of course, determining what is socially unacceptable behavior is extremely problematic and in some cases impossible to account for. What one person may see as socially unacceptable another may not see as a problem.

I see unconditional positive regard as related to the person and not the person's behavior. Thus, I have found in counseling with murderers and other criminals that I actually liked the persons and found that some of the criminal's greatest difficulties were related to others treating him or her like dirt. Often this negative regard was for some behavior that was not directly related to the person who demonstrated the disrespectful attitudes. That is, the person exhibiting the negative regard was not directly affected by the client's behavior. If you steal my car that is one thing. If you steal someone else's car, that is another.

In the attitude of unconditional positive regard the mentor is willing to focus upon the realities of the student's experience no matter what those realities are whether they be anger, sadness, love, or hope. "The therapist [mentor] is willing for the client [student] to be whatever immediate feeling is going on—whether confusion, resentment, fear, anger, courage, love, or pride" (Rogers, 1980, pg. 116). Yet, the mentor values the experiences of the client and is not the carrier of judgment.

Empathy

The mentor is able to experience the feelings and meanings in relationship to the student's experience. Here the mentor enters of the world of the student as if...(Rogers 1961, 1969, 1977, 1980). As if what? First, it is as if the mentor were the student. Seeing the world of the student as the student see it, not as the mentor thinks the student should see it. "What are you angry about that for?" becomes, "I see you are furious that were treated that way."

Second, it is as if the student's world is the mentor's world. If I am sad about something, I find little room for people not grasping my sadness. My sadness often, though not always, makes sense to me. I want my world treated with the respect of it being understood. So the mentor treats the student's world the same way as he or she treats is own world. Perhaps there is a bit of the notion of the Christian exhortation, "Do unto others as you would have them do unto you." So the mentor at least tries to see the world of the student in the same manner as the mentor sees the mentor's own world. "The primary thrust and abiding intent of the therapist [mentor] is to understand the world of each individual from the individual's perspective…and to create an atmosphere of trust that will promote the natural growth process of the individuals …" (Bozarth & Shanks, 1989, pg. 284).

The person-centered mentor endeavors to enter into the world of the individual. I believe this can be done by working to understand and understanding occurs in listening and responding. The empathic response is far more complex than repeating the last words the student says or than paraphrasing. It is often nonverbal. Something the student says makes sense. Its is grasped and assimilated into the mentor's world.

This process toward empathy, I believe, is full of misunderstandings and understandings. Thus, I believe that one should not just share what one understands, but also what one doesn't understand. It is more accurate communication for the student as the student can know when the mentor really understands and is not just believing that the mentor understandings. That is part of being transparent. The student can't "see right through me" (Rogers, 1969) if I don't also let the student see where I am incorrect in my understandings. I believe the student gains confidence that I really understand when I also share what I misunderstand.

Further, if all I do is share my understandings and not my misunderstandings, I cannot really be sure that I have really understood. "Yes, I see," doesn't mean I see anything. I gain confidence in my understanding with the confirmation of the student. I can sharpen my understanding when my course is corrected by the student.

As a mentor I do not dictate the directions for the student. I have input into how we spend our time together and make an impact on the communication, but I don't see it as my place to determine what the student will talk about, or what we will do. I can determine what I am going to talk about and what I am going to do, but I cannot do that for the student. I am willing to share of myself with the student in relationship to the client, but I never assume that anything I do or say will be helpful, appreciated, or interesting to the student. I also don't assume that what I do or say won't be helpful, appreciated, or interesting to the student either. Actually, the last two statements aren't true. I often do make assumptions. However, I usually find out from the student what has been meaningful and helpful about our interactions. Even then, students may not often say if something is helpful or not. Should I make an assumption, without input from the student it is quite often wrong and I have to correct my perceptions.

Using the Rationale: A Mentor's Perspective

The author is a trained counselor and therapist. However, while the principles of the person-centered approach apply to the situation of mentoring, this is not psychotherapy. There may be incidental therapeutic results. Therapy is the reorganization of the self (Rogers, 1961). The client coming for therapy is often coming to restructure who he or she is or at least realign one's self with the self that one truly is. That is always different from individual to individual though we human beings have certain characteristics and types of behaviors in common. However, my characteristics and behaviors are my own, not the reader's.

Mentoring is not about reorganization of the self. It is about engaging another person during a part of his or her pilgrimage through life. The student in the mentoring process may want to change some aspect of himself or herself as a learner, as a person, as a social being, but that is incidental to the mentoring relationship.

Still the approaches for psychotherapy and mentoring are the same. The mentee's goals are different than the goals of the client in psychotherapy.

During our time together, the student makes significant choices about what takes place and addresses our time from his or her resources, one of which is me. For instance, I have requested tours of the school, not because it was an attempt to get the child to do something for me, but because the student has invested time in the school and it is part of the student's world. I learn something about the perceptions of the student from those tours.

As a mentor I am not interested in getting the child to "open-up." I tend to fail in such attempts. By being open myself to the person of the student, I have found that the door opens up to a myriad of experiences and discoveries about who this person is.

I don't assume that a history is important in learning about the student, but the student often tells me about their short lives. These are 2nd to 4th graders, so there isn't a lot of history to tell. But I am often exposed to more information from the student than I can remember about them.

I don't probe about family, but I have learned about brokenness in the home. I have learned where fathers work and live. What has happened to mothers following a divorce. I find out who the grandparents are without ever having to ask probing questions. I have learned where students themselves hurt and what they are interested in as persons.

I am not interested in making students raise issues of the past. Again, what past in these young lives? I am interested in what is taking place here and now (Meador & Rogers, 1984). We can experience this time together, but I am amazed at what I discover as students reflect on their past without being probed and prodded. They may remember a Christmas with family, or a experience with a teacher. Reflections on the past do emerge spontaneously and are often genuine expressions with appropriate meaning for the student in the present.

Application

Bryan

Bryan was a third grader when I first met him. The director of the mentor program and the teacher had encouraged Bryan to give me a tour of the school as an "ice breaker." I checked into the school office and Bryan was paged to come to the office. That page conjured up old images for me as the only times I can remember being paged to the school office was when I was in trouble. Fortunately, Bryan was expecting his mentor to show up and when he arrived we were introduced.

We spoke for a few moments. I don't remember the particulars of the conversation, but I do remember we soon ran out of words. I felt a bit awkward as an adult running out of things to say to a child, but I immediately liked Bryan.

In a few minutes we began the tour. I met the principal and then we went down to the library. There Bryan showed me around the stacks of books making sure I noticed the books about athletes and which one of those he had read. And he also made sure that I noticed the computers and he turned one on pulling up a game he liked about math.

From there we went down the hall and peaked into his class. He waved to the teacher. Other students stared at us as we stood in the doorway. His teacher was busy with the class so I didn't interrupt her other than breaking the attention of the class for a few moments.

We went from there to the gym and then the music room. Bryan told me he sang with the elementary school chorus. He also showed me a couple of percussion instruments he liked to play when Mr. T. passed them out.

Our next stop was the lunch room. Bryan asked me if I would eat lunch with him some time and I agreed to do so in a couple of weeks.

We finished the hallways of the school and went out to the playground.

As we walked about, I discovered Bryan liked to collect baseball cards and liked to read.

With consequence visits I found we didn't talk much. However, Bryan read to me and worked on classroom material which I checked. I was not allowed access to official grades but Bryan reported doing OK in school.

What Bryan seemed to enjoy the most was sorting through baseball cards I brought with me. I let him have the extra cards and there were quite a few. This was tough to do. I am possessive about my possessions. To allow some youngster to have part of my treasure of baseball cards while wondering if he would treasure them as I did was difficult.

But mentoring from the person-centered perspective is not about baseball cards, or things, or even activities. These are incidental to the mentor sharing something of him or her self with the student. What is important are the attitudinal qualities (Bozarth, 1998).

Three years after his mentoring year, I saw Bryan at a middle school band concert. He was playing in the percussion section. I didn't get a chance to say hello as he slipped away to the band room with his drum. I doubt seriously that my handful of contacts contributed to his role in the band. I was proud though that I could make a distant observation of Bryan's pilgrimage and note that I participated in the pilgrimage for a time.

I remember valuing Bryan very much, but I don't remember a lot about him any longer. I remember feeling awkward about silence, but we over came that with classroom assignments he was working on and interacting over the baseball cards. How much of Bryan's world did I enter? Probably not very much. How much did he change? Probably a whole lot more than I was aware of, but mentoring isn't about creating change, it is about encountering a student in a pilgrimage in school and then only getting but a glimpse of that pilgrimage.

Jay

There is one more brief situation that I want to share. I was asked to mentor Jay, a fourth grader, in our new elementary school. I called his teacher to find a time most convenient to his class schedule and for her as his teacher. She welcomed me by anytime. This is pretty standard in the mentoring program here. Ms. Stacy then gave me background material. I prefer not to have such material and she was aware of that. However, she asked if she could share her observations. She told me of his isolation from his fellow students. She said that she behaved inappropriately making a nuisance of himself to classmates, faculty and staff. I thought to myself, "this is my kind of guy." She also said that he probably was not performing up to his potential. "He was warts on his hands," she said and the students don't want to touch him or be touched.

I never really learn from such descriptions and feel they bias the listener. I didn't find him inappropriate. I found him out-going and courteous. He spoke to teachers and students and I never saw him tease another student.

The week that I had conversation with Jay's teacher was involved in a terrible auto accident which took her out of school for the rest of the school year. The following week I met Jay for a tour of the new school and met the substitute teacher who had no idea who Jay was yet. And shortly after that I had lunch with Jay at school.

It is meeting for lunch of which I seek to briefly write.

Jay met me in the principal's office as his class went by for lunch. Since his last name was the first on the roll, he led the class to lunch, as he does everyday. I joined him in line and received lunch. It was ham, green beans, sweet potatoes, and a roll. I picked up a glass of tea and I followed him to the table. I decided to sit across from and asked him if that was OK.

I will not interpret or intellectualize here. The response in one way was small but spoke volumes. He said, "Yes, You can sit there. No one sits there. No one sits here in the seat next to me either." At lunch time with his classmates all sitting at the long table and the teacher sitting with the teachers, Jay sits alone.

I did note above that Jay is not shy. He talked with the students in his class at the table. He spoke clearly to fellow students as they walked by. Not one responded verbally. Several did not even look at him after he greeted them. He knew who they were, but they acted like they didn't even know he was alive.

With that I say no more about Jay. I don't know the other students and I have no idea why they did not speak. I was struck that no one sat next to or across from Jay at lunch. I was also struck by the fact that students Jay knew by name and spoke to did not speak to him when he said hello.

It is here that a portion of person-centered approach for mentoring becomes important. As was pointed out previously, this is not about therapy. It may not even be about change. But what it is about is caring. It is about encountering another where he or she is and engaging that student, that person, even when others may fail to do so for any number of reasons. It is not about what one knows, or what one can find out. It is about respect, understanding, and genuineness.

My experience with Jay was too recent to have the audacity to claim improvement in grades, or reading skills, or other aspects of education. It was too limited by time and frequency to assert that permanent change took place. I repeat that mentoring isn't about facilitating change, though I suspect change takes place. I will say that the interpersonal relationships between Jay and myself were not too limited to make a claim of caring in the midst of estrangement and alienation.

These situations sometimes remind me of an Episcopalian priest I met while I was doing Clinical Pastoral Education at the Rehabilitation Center at Emory University Hospital in Atlanta, GA. Father Garland was racked with arthritis. He was bed ridden with the disease. His fingers and his toes pointed side ways and he lived his life in extreme persistent pain. Yet there he was in a rehabilitation center designed to help people function at their maximum potential. This man would never get out of bed again. Yet, they did therapy on a man who would not physically improve while they turned away younger people away who might improve. Initially I was stunned by the rehabilitation center's willingness to work with a person who clearly would not get better. I even stated that in staff meetings.

I liked the Father Garland, but I didn't see that being a patient at a leading hospital did him any good. Yet he consistently reported that the physical therapy he received diminished his pain during the time he received treatment. He thus felt better during and immediately after the therapy.

His hopeless situation helped me formulate a position of helping. It is not always about restoration, or significant improvement. Sometimes physical and psychological therapy is about being with people in their distress and that this sometimes, though not always, helps a person to feel better.

Thus, I believe that with Jay there was improvement during the mentoring time. He had someone to sit with him a lunch. He had someone in his life who drove all the way over to the school just to see him. I didn't get to do that enough. But I was his mentor and he proudly told people that.

With the person-centered approach, I cannot always argue for improvement at the therapeutic level or the mentoring level. Each situation is so unique and so different that one has trouble determining what improvement is. I don't know if Bryan or Jay are better people for having contact with my version of the person-centered approach. I do feel I got glimpses of who they were. I felt I practiced what I preached. I suspect they are different in some way because we made contact, but I can't prove it.

Conclusion

This is chapter was obviously not a quantitative research based chapter. It is a qualitative researched article with a focus on literature and anecdotal encounters. No case can be presented for the effectiveness of the person-centered approach here. It is however, a care based chapter. The focus is upon an approach to helping, to being of service to students. The chapter therefore finds its integrity not in results, but in the time honored effort to care about others. The students I encountered were often misunderstood, unappreciated, and alienated. If for only the time of the visit they received care in the form of acceptance, understanding, and genuineness, the effort was impactful in ways that no one may be able to measure. No pretense can be made as to improvement in grades, or social interaction as no study was made of such improvement.

At the same time, we also cannot access the extent the students have the "attitudinal qualities" (Bozarth, 1998)) in their lives. Certainly those of us in the person-centered approach have no corner of these qualities. Also no measurement was made as to the level of the "core conditions." However, we do believe that these qualities are essential to growth and change. Thus, in theory, backed by research in the arenas of therapy and counseling, we can assert that students change when they encounter the conditions even in their everyday environments. The teachers, the staff, the fellow students, and even the parents are possible resources for the conditions espoused.

Yet, that the approach exists as a theory suggests that people are either unaware that these qualities are healing, caring, supportive qualities, or they have little confidence that they are. We do live in a quick fix society and the person-centered approach makes no such promise.

Here with the person-centered approach to mentoring we offer care and support. Researchers may be interested in seeking to discover the effectiveness of the approach. It is obvious that this mentor was interested in mentoring, not research.

References

Bower, D. W. (1985). Assumptions and Attitudes of the Rogerian Person-Centered Approach to Counseling: Implications for Pastoral Counseling. Unpublished manuscript, Columbia Theological Seminary, Decatur.

Bower, D. W. (1994). Thwarting self-actualization or fostering self-deactualization: a person-centered perspective. **The Person-Centered Periodical**, 1, 41-49.

Bozarth, J. D. (1985). Quantum Theory and the Person-Centered Approach. **Journal of Counseling and Development**, **64** (3) 179-182.

Bozarth, J. D. (1995). Person-centered therapy: A misunderstood paradigmatic difference? **The Person-Centered Journal**, **2**, (2) 12-17.

Bozarth, J. D. (1996). A theoretical reconceptualization of the necessary and sufficient conditions for therapeutic personality change **The Person-Centered Journal**, **3**, (1) 44-51.

Bozarth, J. D. (1998). Person-centered therapy: A revolutionary paradigm. Ross-On-Wye: PCCS Books

Bozarth, J. D., and Brodley, B. T. (1986). Client-centered psychotherapy: A Statement. **The Person-Centered Journal**, **1**, (3) 262-271.

Bozarth, J. D., and Shanks, A. T. (1989). Person-centered family therapy with couples. **The Person-Centered Journal**, **4**, (3) 262-271.

Brodley, B. T. (1982). **Criteria for making empathic responses in client-centered therapy**. Paper presented at the First International Forum on the Person-Centered Approach, Oaxtepec, Mexico.

Hall, C. S., & Lindzey, G. (1978). **Theories of personality**. New York: John Wiley and Sons.

Jackson, G. E. (1981). **Pastoral Care and Process Theology**. Washington, D.C.: University Press of America.

Lowe, V. (1966). **Understanding Whitehead**. Baltimore: John Hopkins Press.

Meador, B. D., & Rogers, C. R. (1984). Person centered therapy. In R. Corsini (Ed.), **Current psychotherapies** (3rd ed.). (pp. 142-195). Itasca, Illinois: F. E. Peacock Publishers.

Rogers, C. R. (1957). The necessary and sufficient conditions of therapeutic change. **Journal of Consulting Psychology, 21**, 95-103.

Rogers, C. R. (1959). A theory of therapy, personality, and interpersonal relationships, as developed in the client-centered framework. In S. Koch (Ed.), **Psychology: A study of a science: Vol. 3: Formulations of the person and the social context** (pp. 184-256). New York: McGraw-Hill.

Rogers, C. R. (1961). **On becoming a person**. Boston: Houghton Mifflin.

Rogers, C. R. (1969). **Freedom to learn in the 80's**. Columbus: Charles E. Merrill Publishing.

Rogers, C. R. (1977). **On personal power**. New York: Dell.

Rogers, C. R. (1980). **A way of being**. Boston: Houghton Mifflin.

Whitehead, A. N. (1978). **Process and reality: An Essay in cosmology**. Corrected Edition; D. R. Griffin, & D. W. Sherburne (Eds). New York: Free Press.

Person-Centered Politics:
A Personal Pilgrimage

Doug Bower

I have long enjoyed much of the writing style of Carl Rogers. He seems so personal to me. His learnedness appears in his writing, but he doesn't overwhelm readers. His writing is reader friendly, readable (Rogers, 1961, 1977, 1980).

It is not my desire to emulate Rogers. It is my desire to communicate as Doug Bower. Yet, I am consistently prevented from doing so. I have lost count of the number of articles and papers which were rejected as unworthy of publication. It is true that if I edited the documents according to the requests of editors, more of my material would have been published. However, it would not have been my material. It would have been writing that conformed to the expert expectations of an editor or editorial staff.

To me that is the stereotype of politics. Decisions are made elsewhere. The constituent is expected to conform to those decisions, or at least resign one's self to those expectations. Thus involvement is limited to those who are willing to conform or who are willing to try to make change. This politics is in every discipline. It is in medicine, religion, and education.

My intention here is to share something of my experience in politics, the running for public office, involvement in efforts to elect others, or asserting a cause. I hope that in the course of the this paper that a view of politics emerges that recognizes that individuals have political power even if that political power is a minority position.

I ran for public office four times, once for the congress of the United States and three times for the Georgia General Assembly. I was not elected, but I was a winner and have been a winner in politics. Theodore Roosevelt said:

It is not the critic who counts; not the man who points out how the strong man stumbles, or where the doer of deeds could have done them better. The credit belongs to the man who is actually in the arena, whose face is marred by dust and sweat and blood; who strives valiantly; who errs, and comes short again and again; because there is not effort without error and shortcoming; but who does actually strive to do the deeds; who knows the great enthusiasms, the great devotions; who spends himself in a worthy cause, who at the best knows in the end the triumphs of high achievement and who at the worst, if he fails, at least fails while daring greatly, so that his place shall never be with those cold and timid souls who know neither victory nor defeat. (Nixon, 1990, Preface material)

Real Politics in Politics.

I am not clear in my mind how far I should go back in my interest in politics. My first president was Eisenhower. My recollection was that as a child I had warm respectful feelings for him. It was not until I became more learned in history and politics that I discovered there were people who didn't like him, who didn't believe he was a good president (Ambrose, 1983). I cannot say that discovering that others had trouble with Eisenhower altered my own feelings about him. I suspect like the rest of us, he had his weaknesses and his strengths.

I have to put Richard Nixon in my first recollections of politics as well. Here too, I held warm regard for him and did so even through Watergate (Nixon, R., 1990). Naivete' prevailed in my innocence and political thinking.

I would characterize my own initial political pilgrimage as resignation and apparent apathy. I don't remember when I cast my first vote. If I were pressed, I would have to say I cast my first vote when former Georgia governor Jimmy Carter ran for election as president in 1976 (Carter, J., 1982). I had positive images of him was well. I wasn't particularly impressed with his reelection campaign of 1980. Yet, I voted for him as I was afraid that Reagan (Reagan, 1992) would attempt to usher in the kingdom of God by going to Israel's rescue or inciting conflict in the Mideast. It turned out that I was quite please with my attitude during the Reagan administration. I felt secure, safe, and prosperous.

I have deeper recollections of my first active involvement in politics. This involvement took place while I was the associate pastor at the First United Methodist Church in Griffin. I began writing letters to the editor in support of an effort in the community to encourage voters to pass a bond issue to improve school buildings and facilities in Spalding County.

I thought I would receive flack from the members of the church on this issue, but I did not. Any church members who disagree kept those disagreements to themselves. I didn't hear a word from the senior pastor on the issue and he was a person who loved to criticize. That bond passed. I do remember receiving thank-you comments from those supporting the effort, though we were all aware that my efforts were hardly the driving force behind the passage of the bond issue.

Shortly after I moved to Athens, Georgia in 1982 a bond issue concerning education arose there as well. Again I supported the effort. This time I did receive negative feedback. I received a call from a man asking about those who were on fixed income. The conversation initially went well. The issues were discussed with a friendly attitude. Then the man asked me where I was from. "I was born in Niagara Falls, New York," I said. His demeanor changed. He yelled at me over the phone. "You damn Yankees come down here and keep trying to change our education system." He hung up the phone and I was left in my anxiety and guilt for being supportive of an effort to improve education and being a Yankee. It was clear in his initial part of the conversation that the caller disagreed with the bond issue I supported. However, I was traumatized with the condescending nature of the second part of the call after I revealed I was a "Yankee."

Andrew Young for Governor

In 1990, I became interested in the campaign for Georgia governor of Andrew Young former Ambassador to the U.N. under Jimmy Carter, and who had been very active with Martin Luther King, Jr. in the civil rights movement. I volunteered to help with his campaign and made several trips to his campaign headquarters in Athens. I didn't have occasion to meet him, so I supported him based on his reputation. In part I wanted to help get a "black" person elected as the first governor. I thought Mr. Young provided us with an excellent candidate regardless of race.

During that I met a retiree named Betty who had been involved in political campaigns for years. We had a number of enjoyable talks as we held down the fort at Mr. Young's campaign headquarters in Athens. I remember one conversation where she complained that someone on Mr. Young's campaign team in Atlanta came to Athens and chewed out the campaign team for not being aggressive enough. She was hurt and angry over that. It struck me that it didn't sound very motivating. Now it appears to me the expression of an anxious person who was very aware that Mr. Young's campaign was in trouble.

In a later conversation, she told me that it was her last campaign. She said she felt that at her age she didn't need to be so active in politics. I don't know if it was actually her last campaign or not. I remember only seeing her once at a distance a few years later and didn't get to speak with her.

On primary day that year, I volunteered to pick up people to take the polls to vote. On my first and last effort to do so, I went to an apartment to pick up several people. One was a mentally handicapped woman who staggered to the car and sat in the back with her family. However, she urinated on my back seat. I didn't know this until we got to the polls and her family made her get out of the car and go into vote. "You said you wanted to vote," her mother said. "Now get out of the car and go in and vote." The young lady got out of the car and went into the poll site with her pants all wet and urine running down her legs. When they returned, I took them home and then went home myself to clean up the mess. I didn't go back to the campaign headquarters. It was just more than I could handle.

Andrew Young lost his campaign for the Democratic nomination for governor to long term politician and then lieutenant governor, Zell Miller who eventually brought the lottery to Georgia. Actually, the voters brought the lottery to Georgia, Governor Miller and his colleagues just made it possible for the citizens to decide to bring the lottery to Georgia. He was later elected to a second term even though he promised in his first campaign not to run a second term. However, politics was in his blood and he had to. He eventually obtained one of the highest approval ratings as a governor in this history of the state.

Cedar Shoals High School Football Incident: Campaign for an Elected School Board

I have served as unofficial chaplain for the Cedar Shoals High School football program, Athens, Georgia, since 1982. Initially, I offered my services as a registered nurse and gave that up to become chaplain. It has been an enjoyable experience for me over the years and I have only regretted not getting to know the athletes better and having a better mind to remember the names of those I did get to know. I remember faces of those who show up to the games after they graduate, but I can recall only a few of the names.

On the last game of the 1989 season, I was preparing to enter the school complex on my way to the coaching office when one of the football players, Mitch, came up to me and said, "Doc, they took away our victories."

"Your kidding," I said.

I knew at some level he was not kidding. My comment was a statement of shock and disbelief. The team was 8-1 at that point and ranked in the state with eyes upon entering into the play-offs for the state championship. The action of stripping the team of its victories took it out of the play-offs.

I went up to the coaching office where I found the coaches beside themselves in shock, anger, and confusion.

"What happened?" I asked.

"The state association has ruled that we have been playing with an ineligible player," a coach said.

At the beginning of the season, teachers had reevaluated grades on one of the athletes and changed three of his grades. These grade changes made the young man eligible to play.

At this point the situation gets too complex to present here. There were charges that the grades were changed to make the player eligible to play football rather than legitimate changes due to teacher decisions. The Professional Practices Commission was brought in to investigate. Two teachers were placed on probation, the Athletic Director, and the head football coach were fired. In addition the principal was forced to retire early.

The best I could determine from listening to teachers and following reports on the investigation, all the teachers followed established protocol for changing the grades. I was not in a position to determine the motives of the teachers involved. None of them claimed to be changing the grades so the student could play football. Yet, it was clear that his being an athlete put him in a position for someone to notice that he had been wronged by the system. Yet, someone might have noticed that eventually anyway. There was a protocol in place to change grades, and teachers had a right to make changes grades. They argued the changes were justified. It was also clear to me that the teachers believed that the student had been improperly handled causing the poor grades.

After the Professional Practices Commission became involved, it appeared to me that the school superintendent then went on a witch hunt. Heads began to roll. The reaction to the situation seemed to be getting more and more out of control. By following protocol, the grade changes fell into the domain of the administrative office of the school system. They were approved like any other grade changes. Yet, teachers were being threatened. They seemed to be fed to the sharks by the school superintendent.

The investigation demonstrated that the grade changes indeed were allegedly made after established deadlines. Yet, no one in the system said, nor did the computer system itself say, that the grade changes were inappropriate. Thus the grade changes were approved in relationship to established protocol. As far as the coaches were concerned, the students record was corrected and he was eligible to play. Yet, the head coach and the athletic director were treated like they were the one's responsible for the grade changes and they were fired.

With the action of the Georgia High School Athletic Association, and the Professional Practices Commission players, coaches, and supporters at Cedar Shoals were devastated. One of the players from that team is presently coaching at Cedar Shoals. He remains heart broken by what happened to him and the team. I spoke to him again during the 1999 about the incident. His recollections were similar to mine above. He doesn't blame the coaches, but is still hurt that someone along the way didn't forbid those changes. He is still furious that official bodies stepped in and violated the sovereignty of the system here and stripped the team of its victories.

As the school superintendent responded with fierce almost vengeful wrath, I began publicly responding to the punishment that was delved out. Following many of the articles that hit the newspaper, I sent in a letter to the editor. The story was persistent and so was I. A few years later my mentor at the University of Georgia counseling program told me that he was embarrassed for me. Yet, there was something about the dynamics of the school superintendent's involvement that didn't seem in sync. He didn't support his teachers, his coaches, or his principle at Cedar Shoals. He seemed vindictive. One day he called me because of my persistent fussing over the way the situation was being handled. I don't remember what was said, but I do remember feeling defensive and discounted. He seemed to feel unjustly treated. I tried to say to him that was exactly the way his teachers felt. They felt that he didn't understand or appreciate their position and that he was over reacting. He asked me, "What do you want." "Justice," I said. I never heard from him again, but I heard a lot about him.

The way the grade change situation was handled kept drawing attention to the superintendent. I kept feeling like something wasn't right and it wasn't about changing grades. Apparently others felt that way as well. It was not long before the school superintendent and a couple of his lieutenants were charged with mishandling funds for computers. The school superintendent was eventually conflicted of illegal activities. The conviction was later over turned, but a lieutenant went to jail.

While I didn't like the state athletic associations decision, it was set up for this kind of situation. I was not in a position to argue on behalf of Cedar Shoals before the association. Yet, I believe the sovereignty of the teachers who changed the grades was violated by the assumption that they were not acting in good faith. Also the sovereignty of the school system was violated in that its protocol affirmed the grade changes thus allowing the young man to play football.

As heads began to roll, many of us directly and indirectly appealed to the school board to offer some sanity and compassion to the situation. We were met with what we felt was apathy and indifference.

As the tension continued to grow, citizens in the community began seeing the school board as being unanswerable to the community. The members were appointed to the board by the county commissioners and the city governments.

I started hearing calls for an elected school board. And having made several appeals to the school board encouraging them to get the school superintendent to back off and act with some compassion, I felt less and less heard.

So I took a simple initiative. I was not a resident of the county, though I owned property in the county and had a small counseling practice in the county. I was painfully aware that my tax-dollars were being used to support the present system. I placed an announcement in the paper calling for a meeting of citizens who were interested in getting an elected school board. I didn't put my name in it as I didn't feel that as a voter in another county I had the political right to organize such a group. However, since I was a property owner and tax payer, I did feel I had the right to get things started.

Twenty plus people showed up at the initial meeting. I was pleased. They were of course puzzled at not knowing who called the meeting, but they quickly organized and began working to get an elected school board. I was naive as to how the process of this effort would occur. I still am. Far more political actions went on than I was and am aware of. Political hoops had to be jumped through to get a referendum on the ballot. I am sure that it required approval from the state government though I cannot point to the specific documents saying this would be so.

When the referendum was placed on the ballot, 80% of the voters said, "We want to elect our school board members." There was some concern during the campaigning to get this referendum that good citizens would run for the position since it would cost money to do so. This has not been a problem. There have been plenty of interested candidates for the positions.

Very briefly, I would say that a couple of thoughts are important here. First, while I took initiative to get a group going, I did not offer directive actions. This was a citizens' project that evolved based on the participation of more people than I was aware of. It accepted Carl Rogers' notion that was is most personal is most universal (Rogers, 1961). It also supports my basic premise in relationship to democracy that people can be trusted to run the government, that they have vast resources for changing political situations, and if they make a mistake they can and in all likelihood will change it. That does not mean that everyone will like what takes place or trust what takes place.

Campaign against lottery

After having just said that people can be trusted to run the government, I know turn to something that I totally and completely opposed and still oppose, the lottery.

In 1990 seeds were planted to install the lottery here in Georgia. The money was/is to be used for education, mainly for technology, Hope scholarships, and preschool programs. It was an "ends justifies the means" philosophy I have not been able to appreciate.

Unlike the elected school board effort, I cannot claim to feel much impact concerning the antilottery campaign. I supported it mentally and spiritually, but I was never seen as a person who made a difference. I wrote material, prepared a handful of products against the lottery, but was completely dependant on others who opposed the lottery. There were rallies against it. There were no rallies for it. It looked like the forces against the lottery were taking a public position and if one were to gage success for a campaign, I thought public visibility would be a good indicator. It was not. The lottery passed even though I saw no public efforts to support its passage except for some advertisements.

Clearly, the majority of the voters who voted wanted the lottery. I have never felt comfortable about that decision. One, I don't see discarding previously regarded moral standards as being constructive in a society. Instead a I see a society that attempts to overcome years of tradition being wrangled with guilt, shame, anxiety, and confusion and distrust in its attempts to justify behavior that has been poorly regarded for generations. A society just doesn't stop having feelings because it approves a behavior that it once considered wrong.

Second, I saw and still see the dollar signs flashing. This endeavor isn't about education, it has been about profit. Millions of dollars are making it into the pockets of people who espouse the lottery. Education gets a mere pittance of the profit. Those who really profit from the lottery are the providers of equipment, those who are employed to run the operations, those who sell the tickets, and the chief administrators of the lottery.

Also, Georgia after several years of lottery funds being used for education has not seen improvement. Georgia at this writing still ranks 49th in the nation. After all is done, education gets what is left over.

I feel we sold ourselves out to principles that heretofore had been held in poor esteem and actually still are though we have a myriad of rationalizations for justifying the behaviors that surround the lottery.

We are also addicted to the lottery. Take away someone's substance and you get, anger, resentment, confusion, resistance, anxiety, slick rationalizations, and a host of other feelings. When forces seem to mount to do away with the lottery, these very same addictive feelings begin to emerge. A panic of dependency sets in. It already shows up with students who have or might receive "Hope" scholarships. They fear they won't be able to go to college even though C students somehow manage to get through school without "Hope" scholarships.

Addictive behaviors show up in relationship to fears that educational technology will be taken away and leave students somehow maimed and deprived, even though the technology changes so fast that it virtually impossible to keep up financially with the changes.

Money is in essence thrown away on programs and equipment that just about the time people discover how to use them, they have to buy new equipment and software. There seems to be little trust in people and their natural resources. The trust has shifted to money and technology. If we just have lottery money we can excel. I don't see security, confidence, or even actualization of the educational program emerging.

Campaigns for Congress & State House

In November or December of 1991, I began seriously contemplating running for public office. Not having run before and still feeling very tentative about running, I decided not to run in a race with an incumbent.

"Incumbents always have the edge," I thought to myself. I didn't see that a person without experience would do well against an incumbent. I have sense seen that is not always true. Yet, that is what I mistakenly believed at the time.

I looked locally first, then to the state General Assembly races. Each had an incumbent. Then Doug Barnard, then Congressman for the 10th District in Georgia, announced he would no longer seek office. A couple of factors came into play. First, here was a race without an incumbent.

Second, the premise that what is most personal is most universal kept running through my mind. Politics and government belongs to "regular" citizens. It should not be left in the hands of the elite. The elite I defined as those who could personally finance a campaign, or could influence enough people to give money to a campaign.

Third, I had felt and still felt that politics should be about people, not about money. I find spending large amounts of money on a campaign an atrocity. I tend to believe that a politicians who believes he or she should spend and waste a lot of money on a campaign, will do so with taxpayers' dollars once elected. I have seen nothing to change that and much to support it. For instance one politician I saw disclosure forms on held staff meetings in expensive hotels putting up campaign staffers for three or four nights. Another held meetings in country clubs. The list of spending habits is endless. If one has the mind set that I can't run a campaign without throwing money around, I can't see how one can find a way to run government on less money. Creativity doesn't cost a cent. It is ingrained in people.

Fourth, I also felt that if I was bothered by the spending habits of government, there were others who were also bothered by those spending habits. While I never came close to being elected, a high percentage of people whom I interacted with believed this. It was clear though that the tremendous numbers of voters I didn't meet didn't vote according to that conviction. That meant, that those who believed as I did sought me out and made it easy for me to meet them. Or it meant that voters had no confidence that the myth about money could be broken so they supported the status-quo. The most logical position was that I didn't make enough of an impact on potential voters to get their attention and thus got my political rear kicked.

I brought a great deal of naivete into the campaign. I actually believed that people would read the newspapers and would take political ads seriously. I also actually believed that once I announced that my phone would start ringing off the hook, not from supporters, but from interested citizens, newspaper writers, and news casters who were seeking information. It didn't happen. My announcements and my efforts were for the most part met with silence.

I knew my efforts were in trouble not because I actually ran the low budget campaign I wanted to run, I practiced what I preached, I knew I was in trouble because I was never attacked. I also had trouble getting county chairpersons to contact me, calls weren't returned, messages weren't clarified, and I never once got an invitation to attend a county meeting during my first campaign. I had to take all the initiative.

Fifth, I also wanted to run a positive campaign characterized by respect for my fellow candidates and certainly by respect for the citizens. Imagine politicians respecting one another. I did it. We did it. For the most part, the five Democrats, and five Republicans were very respectful of one another. I feel more than confident that my own attitude helped the other candidates to run positive races. Now when the Democratic primaries were over, some mud started to get thrown around between the two former front runners. Even then this mud slinging didn't take place to any great extent publicly and quickly disappeared.

The reality set in during the campaign. Either only a handful of persons were listening, or 95% of the voters were unimpressed. Perhaps in my own arrogance, I felt I should have been elected. However, as far as I could tell I was not identified as someone who really believes that government wastes and spends too much money perpetuating itself.

In the process of running for office, I certainly found politics was not the dreadful monster that we have painted it to be. I was impressed by all the candidates that ran for congress in the 10th District that year. However, I had a sense who was most likely to win even though I conducted no surveys. That was going to either Congressman Ben Jones who had once had a role in the TV series Dukes of Hazard, or Don Johnson who had a strong political family in Northeast Georgia. I was surprised that there was no run off in the Democratic primary however.

Still it was traumatic to run and lose even though I figured that being new to politics and not being particularly socially assertive (shy), that I wouldn't receive the party's nomination.

Yet I was encouraged because I rationalized in my own mind I started out with only one vote, mine, and wound up with 5% of the democratic vote on low name recognition and upon spending less than $5000. I was completely in the hands of the voters.

I was quite blown away when a couple of weeks after the primaries I received a little note card from then Secretary of State Max Cleland simply saying, "I'm proud of you." Tears starting flowing when I read it and I still can't tell that story without tears coming to my eyes even as I wrote this paragraph.

I have since ran for the State House as a Republican three times. I haven't found the issues have changed. Government still spends too much money and gives little back spending its money to perpetuate its own interests. Education here in Georgia still flounders at 49th in the nation. Crime is still a problem with the perception that criminals need to serve the full sentences while it would cost us more to house prisoners. There is also the reality that the prison systems themselves are so riddled with oppressive behaviors that even those who work in them feel oppressed and overwhelmed by the system.

I faired better in my efforts to run for the State House. However, with the 1998 campaign after figuring I had more name recognition, that I was on the right side of the issues calling for less government, less spending, campaign finance reform, a change in course for education, I received a lower percentage of the votes that I ever had in an election.

This left me flabbergasted and bewildered. I deliberately choose to run low budget campaigns attempting to put my trust in the will of the people. Then I start abandoning that by finding ways to get people to vote for me. When I do this I am at my most miserable state as a candidate. I give up the trust and start worrying.

Still one needs money to get the word out. Direct mail is not inexpensive. Newspapers give the best rates, but my confidence that a newspaper ad reaches the people who vote is low. With direct mail I can target voters. But I haven't been able to afford to send out three or four pieces of mail to 8000 voters. Somewhere there has to be a balance between spending $40,000 on a campaign and $5000. The question at the writing is doing I have the patience and persistence to pull this off. And the second is, "Maybe the reality is that no matter what Doug Bower does as a candidate, the voters have not been, nor will they ever be interested in my philosophy of trust in people verses money.

A recent campaign of sorts concerning the pending arrival of a company seeking to develop an old granite pit becoming a gravel pit captured my attention. I informally joined an effort to resist its arrival. I had been hearing from people who living near the project did not want its presence. I wrote the following letter to the editor expressing my views and positions.

Clearly it reflects my doubts that the gravel project would benefit the county.

I am quite concerned about a growing threat to the integrity of life-style in Oglethorpe County.

This is my home. My family and I chose to be here and remain here. Both my wife, and I moved around a lot and never really had roots established. The closest I came to such roots was growing up in the Bradenton-Sarasota area of Florida. Some of my acquaintances have moved to Georgia because of the growth there.

I have now lived in Oglethorpe County longer than any place. We chose to live here because of the country setting, and the friendly people. It is far more attractive to get up in the morning and hear the birds singing, and the wind blowing rather than tires squealing and the noise of traffic. The aroma of honey suckle beats the aroma of a polluted air any time. It is far more important to me to know my neighbors than to not have a clue who there are. I consider this county an oasis in a desert of "progress."

I fear the proposed arrival of the M & M project poses a major threat to the life style of the county. If I thought the M & M project would improve the life style of Oglethorpe County, I would be glad to support the endeavor and wouldn't write this letter.

If I wanted "progress" of the kind that M & M appears to be offering, I would have returned to Florida years ago. When I visit my old home in Florida, I see a nearby creek so polluted there is not a shiner, or a bass to be seen. I see a road that I cannot even cross without endangering my life. I used to be able to ride a bicycle 3 miles to Oneco and not see a car on Saturday morning on that same road.

I could have also stayed in Clarke County where I have many friends. There is a lot of "progress" there. There is also a lot of chaos there. It has a higher pollution index. There is more noise there. The traffic is getting crazier and crazier. The school system has been struggling, though it seems to be improving thanks to dedicated staff. Still some of Clarke County's best teachers are making their way to Oglethorpe County to teach.

Proponents for the arrival of M & M have said it's project would offer jobs to residents of Oglethorpe County. I have great doubts about this. The people who handle their equipment need training. The company undoubtedly has a fleet of vehicles and trained personnel already. They won't need to train folks as they, in all likelihood, have a waiting list for their positions. They may need some folks to do the dirty work, but I am sure that will be kept to a minimum. Dirty work generally doesn't generate profit.

Proponents also say we need to extend our tax base and get tax relief for the property owner. I am always for that. However, my mother, who still lives in Florida, has a postage stamp of a piece of property in Manatee County. Every time there is progress her property tax goes up, not down. And there is a lot of progress there. She is paying as much in taxes for her small piece of property as I do for my 5 acres of land and house here in Oglethorpe County. So, we are getting a tax break. Our taxes are lower here than any place I have lived. I have lived in Spalding County, Gwinnett County, and Dekalb County. Increasing industry does not bring lower taxes, it brings higher taxes.

We moved here to improve our life style and we did. Living in Oglethorpe County is a step up from where I have lived, not a step down.

I often get the impression though that some of the residents here think that we live in a second rate county. They apparently believe it will somehow get better if we get a lot more trucks pounding on our roads, if we increase industry and raise the pollution index (I noted in the Athens Banner/Herald that Oglethorpe County did not even show up on a recently published story on major polluters). The greatest pollution risk here is spring pollen which subsides greatly when spring is completed.

If M & M arrives, it will indeed be pounding our roads with heavy trucks. The tax-payers of the county will have to pay for that pounding. Our car tags will increase as well as the property taxes. No doubt sales taxes will have to increased. As other industries arrive, taxes will go up to supply them with water, roads, and services. Progress is a consuming monster that eats tax dollars while generating profits for people who don't live in this county and don't really care about the county.

The bottom line is money. If M & M didn't think it could make a buck, it wouldn't be looking at Oglethorpe County. Yet, very few people in Oglethorpe County will profit from M & M being here. Quite a few will be directly adversely affected. Their privacy will be disrupted. Their peace will be altered. Taxes will go up, and the land will be further scarred.

People will be left feeling further discouraged that what they want doesn't matter. Then we will be asking why people don't get involved.

I have no reason to believe that the gravel project is being set up for the benefit of Oglethorpe County. I also have no reason to believe that many of the local proponents of the project will directly or even indirectly benefit from the project. Therefore I am puzzled that there is any local support for the project at all. The project will bring consequences that we will be paying for long after it is finished. It will leave us with unkept promises, higher taxes, inconveniences on our roads, increased traffic, inconveniences to neighbors, and a more deeply scarred tract of land. Crime rates in growing areas increase, school systems decline, and the attitudes of the citizens becomes less compassionate.

Our desire for progress does not mean that we need to succumb to just any new industry. Our situation is not desperate.

I like this oasis called Oglethorpe County. I am only interested in improving it. I have seen no evidence that the gravel project of M & M will improve Oglethorpe County. (Bower, 1999)

I received a call from an irate woman who dressed me down for my attitude of resisting change in the county. I have been cussed out in such calls. The woman did not go that far. She called the people of the county low-lives, discredited the local school system as being of poor quality, said there was too much marijuana growing and drug dealing in the county, said that law enforcement was terrible, and that taxes were too high. In regards to the taxes, she said she didn't get any services for the taxes she paid. Even though I told her I was pleased with where I lived, she told me that I should live somewhere else, and no it wasn't that I should go to hell, at least she didn't say that verbally. We were clearly on the opposite sides of the issue and for what seemed to be the exact same reason. She wanted to keep taxes lower. I wanted lower taxes. While she said she wanted improvement in law enforcement. I wanted improvement in law enforcement, but I have not felt law enforcement is terrible. Clearly, we were concerned about crime which I felt and still feel increases in rate at a greater rate than the population increases. We were both concerned about education. If anything brought the woman close to cursing it was when she began to discredit education. I was very pleased with education though improvements are always necessary. That the school system ranked high in the state and has won numerous awards doesn't make it perfect, but does say people in the system have integrity. One of her parting shots to me was that one of the reasons I lost my bid for the state house was that I was closed to growth in the county. I don't doubt that, if one person perceived that others believed that too. However, when I analyzed my defeat, it was clear that I was defeated by a very powerful and wonderful black turnout at the polls. Analysis across the state which held up especially in Greene County and Putnam County showed that 90-95% of the Afro-American voters voted for Democrats. I was dismayed that the party of anti-slavery, emancipation, "Negro Suffrage," the party of Lincoln, got itself branded as being made up of White Racists. I was proud that the Black community joined together to protect its interests, but I suffered the consequences by association with the Georgia Republicans.

Finally, the woman had enough of fussing at me, and disagreeing with me. She couldn't grasp my position. I couldn't support hers. I remain convinced of my points in my letter-to-the editor.

The occasion left me shaken. My heart started skipping beats periodically for 3 or 4 hours afterward. I obsessed about the interaction. When I first started speaking of the call to my family, there energy sky rocked. I felt anxious and guilty for expressing my position publicly.

I am not at all convinced that the woman felt heard, though I felt I heard her. I believe she didn't feel heard because I shared my opposite views. For instance, she claimed that the project would improve taxes, I shared with her my experience in other areas where taxes went up to make projects possible. I also had children in the school system, knew many teachers, principals, and staff, and had seen reports concerning the school system. While I did not point that out to her when she discredited the school system, I am convinced that since I did not really agree with her that she did really feel heard.

I close this section wondering about the obsession of hearing others. I in no way tried to shut this woman up. In fact, I heard a lot that I really didn't want to hear. I really didn't want to feel put down and I didn't want my position discredited. However, no one else has the obligation to adhere to my values in the Person-Centered Approach. I did prize the woman's audacity to call me at home and fuss at me. I was very much aware of the intensity of the feelings which seemed to me be dismay, anger, and close to rage. I didn't want to hear put-downs of the county, the schools, the people, the law enforcement agencies. I especially didn't want to feel guilty that I may not have heard this woman. And I certainly didn't want to feel the awful empty feeling I felt after she hung up saying, "Have a good evening." She didn't call me that I might have a good evening. And I didn't have a good evening. I am convinced that she didn't either. In this, I was empathic. My feelings were mine, but they said something about what the woman felt. By the way, she didn't tell me who she was. Caller ID gave me her number and I had the technology in my office to find where the call came from. However, it seemed more important to allow this woman her anonymity, and certainly not to invade her privacy. She said what she wanted to say, though like myself she may have other thoughts that popped into her mind after hanging up.

This is Person-Centered politics.

Principles

Carl Rogers (1997) wrote:

Politics in present-day psychological and social usage, has to do with power and control: with the extent to which person desire, attempt to obtain, possess, share, or surrender power and control over others and/or themselves. It has to do with the maneuvers, the strategies and tactics, wigging or unwitting, by which such power and control over one's own life and others' live is sought and gained—or shared or relinquished. It has to do withe locus of decision-making power: who makes the decisions which, consciously or unconsciously, regulate or control the thoughts, feelings, or behavior of others or oneself. It has to do with effects of these decisions and these strategies, whether proceeding from an individual or a group, whether aimed at gaining or relinquishing control upon the person himself, upon others, and upon the various systems of society and its institutions.

In sum it is the process of gaining, using, sharing or relinquishing power, control, decision-making. It is the process of the highly complex interactions and effects of these elements as they exists in relationships between persons, between a person and a group, or between groups. (pp. 4-5)

In the extreme the negative kind of politics would be represented by the likes of Hitler, Stalin, and others of their brand of government. However, the model shows up in the Church, at work, at school whenever people are seen as having to be manipulated and controlled.

Rogers (1986) also wrote:

> ...Seeing the human organism as essentially positive in nature—is profoundly radical. It flies in the face of traditional psychoanalysis, runs counter to the Christian tradition, and is opposed to the philosophy of most institutions, including our educational institutions. In psychoanalytic theory our core is seen as untamed, wild, destructive. In Christian theology we are "Conceived in sin," and evil by nature. In our institutions the individual is seen as untrustworthy. Persons must be guided, corrected, disciplined, punished, so that they will not follow the pathway set by their nature. (p. 127)

The danger now is power bashing. With that danger I believe comes the danger of self righteous indignation concerning power politics. Yet, there are differences in attitude if not substance and I will attempt to capture some of the essence of Person-Centered politics.

The basic premise of Person-Centered politics is this, citizens can be trusted to run the government. In fact, the people are the government. I believe that democracy is intended to manifest a model of trust. The trust is based on ability or capability. That is, democracy holds the position that the people have the capabilities and resources to govern themselves and make political decisions. The ability to govern does not rest in a "blood-line" handed down through the ages, but is related to a myriad of psychosocial tangibles. Some of which are presented in the "Declaration of Independence:

We hold these truths to be self-evident, that all men are created equal, that they are endowed by their Creator with certain unalienable rights, that among these are life, liberty and the pursuit of happiness. That to secure these rights, governments are instituted among men, deriving their just powers from the consent of the governed,- That whenever any form of government becomes destructive of these ends, it is the right of the people to alter or to abolish it, and to institute new government, laying its foundation on such principles and organizing its powers in such form, as to them shall seem most likely to effect their safety and happiness.

The element of trust is also inherent in the Preamble of the United States Constitution.

WE THE PEOPLE of the United States, in Order to form a more perfect Union, establish Justice, insure domestic Tranquility, provide for the common defense, promote the general Welfare, and secure the Blessings of Liberty to ourselves and our Posterity, do ordain and establish this Constitution for the United States of America.

I don't want to sound idealistic here. I am not trying to say that the people won't hurt one another. Racial prejudice, murder, lying, political corruption, and other painful realities litter the history of democracy. I am saying that the people are capable of making decisions which effect their lives politically. If those decisions backfire and the consequences are adverse to the society, then those in the society are in a position to change them with their votes, the donations, and the expressions of their opinions.

This country was founded (Peterson, 1970) in a period of history in which despots ruled the leading countries of the day and the people were subjected to that rule (Locke, 1698; Payne, 1791; Burke, 1740). If that leadership was benevolent, then such subjection may have seemed acceptable. If not, then it may have been an intolerable time. I am thinking of the myths of Robin Hood which were written in part to capture the difference between two despotic extremes.

I also submit that democracy creates its own twist to the above despotic scenario and thus has a negative impact on trusting the people. Democracy falls short when the minority is expected to adhere to the will of the majority and even promote the will of the majority. While the concept of democracy is not new, its practice is. The reality is that distrust, manipulation, and other forms of despotism remain.

However, I am convinced that the trust of the person has emerged slowly out of distrust. It has only been recently in history that women, and minority groups have even been allowed to vote. That emergence has been met with resistance through the centuries. Even the early forms of democracy were limited to select individuals. Yet, perhaps that resistance grumbled greatly with the establishment of our own country. "Freedom had been hunted round the globe; reason was considered as rebellion; and the slavery of fear had made men afraid to think." (Paine, p. 6)

So I submit that the people have not always used this trust well having hurt one another, and having been engaged in an ongoing battle for freedom, a freedom that can only truly emerge when an element of trust exists.

O ye that love mankind, yet that dare oppose not only the tyranny, but the tyrant, stand forth! Every spot of the old world is overrun with oppression. Freedom hath been hunted around the globe. Asia, and Africa, have long expelled here.—Europe regards her like a stranger, and England hath given her warning to depart. O! Receive the fugitive and prepare in time an asylum for mankind." (Paine, 1791, p. 39).

Democracy is the attempt to provide that asylum, and asylum based on trust of persons to join together to govern themselves making their own political mistakes, their own political advances, and establishing their own political directions.

The Role of the Person-Centered Politician

I claim here that person-centered politics is based on empathy. In person-centered politics there is an openness to the "will" of the people. There is sensitivity to the desires, hopes, and aspirations of the voters on a variety of issues. The person-centered politician attempts to discover what the will of the people is, by entering into their worlds. This can be done by face-face interactions, participating in forums, and conducting surveys or taking polls.

However, having run for political office I attempted to be open to the "wills" of the people. Yet, the reality is that even by taking polls, one cannot be certain what the will of the people is. A simple majority may say it wants lower taxes and less government spending. That potentially still leaves 50% less 1 voter who disagree or who haven't decided on issues surrounding lower taxes and less government spending. This meant there was a conflict of "will" among the voters.

I also have to say that it was extremely difficult to determine with confidence what the will of the voters and citizens is. It was easy to hear the voices of those who expressed themselves about an issue that I disagreed with. As I campaigned, I was convinced from my research that I was congruent with perhaps 60% of the voters, and 90% of those who spoke to me. Yet, when the election over, the best I ever did was get about 34% of the vote. I am convinced that people who believed what I believed sought me out, those that did not for the most part kept quiet. They sought out my "opponent." I am also convinced that while I had hoped to find unbiased sources of research, I did not find it.

I felt I did hear those who agreed with me and I certainly felt I heard those who did not. I believe I was open to the opinions of others, but people were reluctant to express contrary ideas to me. Those who did were often hostile and insulting.

I remember meeting a member of the KKK in a restaurant who bitterly complained of the demise of the KKK. He told me the reason for that demise was that there "are no longer enough good Christian men" around to belong to the KKK. Such a position is so foreign to my way of thinking that I cannot entertain it. Yet, I was so fascinated that I actually was listening to a person who openly proclaimed once being a member of the KKK, that I discovered a perspective I had never seen up close and first hand before.

Transparency to the People: Genuineness

The person-centered politician is dedicated to being transparent. It is not a dedication to winning. It is a dedication to reveal as much of the politician's beliefs and ideals as possible within the limits of public campaigning and advertising. For instance on the issue of lower taxes and less government spending, I think the government spends and wastes too much of the tax-payers' dollars. It has become too bureaucratic and cumbersome. It often ties itself up with red tape and loop holes in its own policies. Yet, there are those who support large government and higher taxes to support that government. Their fears include the loss of jobs among government workers, loss of contracts to the private sector thus affecting employment in the private sector, and the loss of aid to those in need. That there is government waste means that waste is spent on people and products who in turn pay taxes because they have a job for the government or for a private business that has a contract to supply a product.

My own position if I had been elected would have been to work toward downsizing government, lowering taxes, and cutting waste. My feeling remains that the tax payer would keep his or her hard earned money and decide for him or her self what to do with that money. That decision would be either to spend the money to buy a product or service. The money spent would generate more taxes at each level it was spent. Or the decision would be to save it. In which case the money would be lent to someone who would spend it. Thus it would generate taxes at each level that it was spent. Or the decision would be to give it away. Again it would be used for products and services which are produced by someone who was employed who would spend it, save it, or give it away. The cycle goes on and on and generates tax dollars all along the process of circulating.

The point here is not what the tax payer wants, but is the articulating the politicians position so the voters have a good look at the politicians position, or at least enough of a glimpse of the politician's stance to make a voting decision. Thus the person-centered politician needs to be transparent so the voters can decide. It is my position that politicians who are ambiguous about their positions are in part locked into winning their "race" rather than being open to helping the voter decide. In this the person-centered politician needs to be open to whatever direction the voters decide to take (Rogers, 1951). I believe this openness allows the voters to make more informed decisions, but it is not possible if the politician is wrapped up in winning and telling the voters what they want to hear so the politician can get elected.

Yet, part of this issue may be truly hearing the voters and changing one's behavior to attempt to carry out the will of the voters. During my campaigning I heard much criticism of politicians and leaders who bended with the will of the voters. "You can't let the voters dictate what you are doing." Why not? Is not the politician supposed to represent the people?

At the same time, if the voters want the government to drop atomic bombs on Russia to obliterate it, should the politician give into that desire. I wouldn't. I fall back here on transparency and the strength to stand up for one's beliefs. Perhaps these thoughts here may seem like a contradiction. I look at that in part as the ability of a person to keep his or her act together under a variety of circumstances. To stand one's ground if you will. But I also look at it as having the courage and strength to change one's mind on an issue. Often it is reported in the newspapers and used in debates, that a politician changing his or her mind it lying or being wishy washy. I saw a segment of a discussion on television between Bill Bradley and John McCain on December 16 of 1999. Instead of addressing their own opponents, Bradley addressed issues concerning George Bush, Jr., and McCain addressed issues concerning Al Gore. Gore was accused on vacillating on the issues. He was said to have been anti-abortion, and then became pro-choice. Several other changes in positions were brought up. One statement was that Gore didn't know what he wanted to believe. While I am not an Al Gore fan, is it possible that Al Gore has enough integrity to change his mind on issues given new evidence, or is it possible that he is willing to overlook his own position to respond to the majority of people who hold a position that is contrary to his own.

There has to be a balance between revealing one's position, adjusting it to reflect the desires of the people, and at the same time standing firm in principles that may come in conflict with the will of the people from time to time.

High Regard of the People: Acceptance

In this, the person-centered politician is in a position to hold all taxpayers in high regard. Whether, they are in agreement with the politicians position or not. Can the person-centered politician accept the vote with the realization that he or she helped the voters decide by being transparent, and that the voters said "no, we want the other person to represent us?"

After my run for the democratic nomination for the 10th District Congressional seat in Georgia, 1992, I received a card in my mail box. It was from Secretary of State, Max Cleland. The card simply said, "I am proud of you." The tears flowed when I read that card and still do when I tell the story. I didn't think anybody had noticed my effort.

Max Cleland was invited to speak at the Kiwanis Club of Athens a year or so later. I am a member of that club and was giving the uplift that day. I told that story. And of course, tears came to my eyes as I told the ending. As I walked by Max Cleland he gave me a hug with his remaining arm. He lost an arm and two legs in the Vietnam conflict. Then when he got up to the podium, he looked at me and said: "This reminds me of a story. A politician got up in front of his supporters after losing an election. Stoically he said, 'The voters have spoken. Damn.'" Something is missing from the writing of this story, but we all laughed.

I don't want it to seem that the person-centered politician is immune to the pain of not winning by being open to what the voters decide. It was not fun to run for public office having a sense that I wasn't going to win and it wasn't fun to look at the returns and see that I got my political rear-end kicked. Yet, each time I felt that the overwhelming percentage voters had said, "no, we don't want you, we want the other person." While that didn't feel good to me. It was clear that the voters wanted the other person. Damn!

It hurt to lose the campaigns and not gain the trust of the voters. After my first campaign, I patted myself on the back for getting 5% of the votes for nomination as the democratic candidate for Congress. It pleased me that I was the nominee, by default, as the republican candidate for the Georgia state house. Yet, when I got blown away in the elections three times, it was traumatic. Still my faith in the voters did not waver. I am convinced they did not want to vote for me. I didn't represent the ideals of a majority of the voters. Sure, I wish I did, but I wasn't going to assume a role, an identity that I didn't like in order to get elected. I felt traditional politicians were and are too wrapped up in building financial war chests so they can win. I see too much money being wasted on campaigns and believe that politicians who waste their supporters money getting elected will waste the tax-payers' money once they are elected. While I think it is important to hear differing perspectives, I don't believe in politicians who speak out of both sides of their mouths. Deception troubles me. I believe the voters deserve openness, respect and trust.

References

Ambrose, S. E. (1987). **Eisenhower** (Vols.. 1-2). Norwalk, Connecticut: The Easton Press

Bower, D. W. (1990, April). Letter to the Editor. **Oglethorpe Echo.**

Burke, E. (1790). **Reflections on the revolution in France.** Reprinted in the Classics of Liberty Library. New York: Gryphon Editions, 1992.

Carter, J. (1982). **Keeping faith; Memoirs of a president.** Norwalk, Connecticut: The Easton Press

Locke, J. (1698). **Two treatises of government.** Reprinted in The Classics of Liberty Library. New York: Gryphon Editions, 1992.

Nixon, R. (1990). **In the arena.** Norwalk, Connecticut: The Easton Press

Paine, T. (1791). **Common sense.** Reprinted in The Classics of Liberty Library. New York: Gryphon Editions, 1992.

Paine, T. (1791). **Rights of man: Part the Second.** Reprinted in The Classics of Liberty Library. New York: Gryphon Editions, 1992.

Peterson, M. D. (1970). **Thomas Jefferson and the New Nation.** London: Oxford University Press. Reprinted by The Easton Press: Norwalk, Connecticut, 1987.

Rogers, C. R. (1951). **Client-centered therapy.** Boston: Houghton Mifflin.

Rogers, C. R. (1961). **On becoming a person.** Boston: Houghton Mifflin.

Rogers, C. R. (1977). **On personal power.** New York: Dell

Rogers, C. R. (1980). **A way of being.** Boston: Houghton Mifflin.

Rogers, C. R. (1986). Rogers, Kohut, And Erickson: A Personal Perspective on Some Similarities and Differences, **Person-Centered Review** 1, (2), 125-140.

Reagan, R. (1992). **An American life.** Norwalk, Connecticut: The Easton Press.

Using Intergenerational Resources With Adult Incest Clients

Marlene M. Kuskie

The taboo of talking about incest has been lifted in recent years. Counselors are seeing more clients who are survivors of incestuous sexual abuse. Sexual abuse may not be the presenting concern that brings the client to the counselor's office, but the person-centered relationship provides an environment of trust and openness which allows the client to talk about experiences that have often been denied or repressed for years. Estimates are that one out of every four females has been sexually abused before the age of 18 (Russell, 1986) and that one in ten females is a survivor of incest. (Since the largest number of survivors are female, hereafter the feminine pronoun will be used to refer to the client.) Counselors need to be able to recognize the dynamics of incest and how incest can affect development and then be able to co-create with the client changes to enhance the client's growth and development to becoming a more fully functioning person.

There are many resources for the counselor to consult concerning sexual abuse (Bass & Davis, 1988; Courtois, 1989; Courtois & Watts, 1982; Faria & Belohlavek, 1984; Joy, 1987; Finkelhor, 1984; Mayer, 1983; Poston & Lison, 1989). These resources provide valuable insights concerning the dynamics of sexual abuse and some interventions. But the counselor often continues to struggle to help the client grow beyond the blaming of self, guilt and taking responsibility for the incest experiences.

When incest is the issue, the family frequently is of little help or can be a negative influence in therapy. By encouraging the client to develop an intergenerational relationship with a person whether a child or an older adult outside the family, the relationship can become the catalyst for the client to experience acceptance/support from another so that the positive self-actualizing potential of the client may be realized (Kirschenbaum, 1979).

Dynamics of Incest

Incest is one of the results of disruptive, intergenerational family dynamics (Herman, 1981; Meiselman, 1978; Rosenfeld, Nadelson, Krieger & Backman, 1979; Summit, 1983). The incestuous family has interactional/communication patterns that perpetuate denial and the secret of incest. The lack of acceptance and incongruence of the family makes it particularly helpful for the survivor to be helped by a person-centered counselor. A person-centered counselor provides a fertile environment that can allow the survivor to experience a full range of emotions and will feel supported in challenging attitudes and behaviors that have grown from the abuse but are now hindering the client from whole living (Rogers, 1978). Common characteristics of the incestuous family that prevent other family members from helping the survivor are: role reversal between mother and daughter (Bessett, 1985; Mrazek & Bentovim, 1981); enmeshment between the survivor and perpetrator concerning feelings for and against each other (Courtois & Sprei, 1988; and Saunders, Murphy & McClure, 1987); chaotic interactions that prevent the survivor from trusting other family members (Hoagwood & Stewart, 1989); and rigid patriarchal control in the family (Herman, 1981; Summit & Kryso, 1978). The family often perceives the survivor as the problem, not the perpetrator. The family's problem-solving pattern did not address the survivor's needs and boundaries when the abuse occurred, and change probably has not occurred since that time.

Meiselman (1978) and Summit (1983) stated that it is extremely difficult to isolate the effects of incest from other dysfunctional family issues and that the survivor is often more disturbed by the reactions of the adult members of the family to disclosure of the secret than the actual effects of the sexual activity per se. Thus, the counselor must address and attempt to understand the whole person and all the accompanying feelings, thoughts and behaviors. The previous cited studies suggest that incest is an inter-generational family pattern that makes therapeutic intervention using intergenerational family resources very difficult and the use of intergener-ational resources from the community have a better potential for aiding the healing process.

To better understand how nonfamial intergenerational resources may be helpful, it is important to understand the symptoms that bring the client to the counselor's office. The client may try to deny the effects of the experience(s) but may have any of the following symptoms that can be indicative of sexual abuse: aversion to sex; flashbacks to the molestation experience(s); problems with sexual arousal and orgasm; negative attitudes such as revulsion; fear and powerlessness towards their sexuality; isolation and interpersonal problems particularly in the marital relationship; anger, hostility, fear or overvaluation of men; over sexualization of relationships; chemical abuse; self- destructive behaviors and suicidal tendencies; feel-ings of shame and guilt; low self-esteem; grief and depression; vulnerabil-ity to other forms of abuse; mistrust and suspicion; nightmares and sleep disturbances; phobias and obsessions/compulsions; hypervigilance; a need to control or dominate; and an inability to cope with life's stresses (Finkelhor & Browne, 1985; Jehu, Gazan & Klassen, 1985; Russell, 1986). In the person-centered counseling relationship of genuineness, acceptance and empathy where the counselor can understand and focus on the vast potential of strength and courage that the client has already exhibited (Rogers, 1980), the symptoms of depression (anger directed at the self), suicide attempts, guilt, low-self esteem, chemical abuse and interpersonal difficulties can be set aside to discover the client's feelings and desire for change. It is this reservoir of courage, i.e. that client has responded to life and continued to grow in spite of fear, that empowers the client to embark upon a journey of growth and change that can be very rewarding but also very painful.

The feelings that often keep the client from drawing upon her own inner strength are guilt and self-blame which result in depression (Gelinas, 1983; Janoff-Bulman & Frieze, 1983; Miller & Porter, 1983). Janoff-Bulman (1979) attributed the emergence of guilt and self-blame as a coping mechanism the survivor develops. These coping strategies allow the client to feel that there was some control over the situation, i.e. if the client feels guilt, then at least she could have said "no" and had some control in the situation. Most often the client attributes the cause of the abuse to unchangeable characteristics in herself and that it was her fault, which in-turn frequently causes additional self-deprecation, hopelessness and powerlessness. Even though the counselor and the community-at-large may verbally reassure the client that the incest experience(s) were not her fault, the client continues to feel responsible. The client views the experiences from an adult perspective and has suppressed the vulnerability, decision-making process, thoughts and feelings of being a child.

Development of the Survivor

Piaget & Inhelder (1969) labeled the cognitive development of a child during the ages 5-11 as preconcrete operational and concrete operational. The child at these ages is able to cognitively perform certain actions on objects or events as long the child can perceive cause and effect in a very concrete manner. In addition, egocentricity in the child's thinking causes the child to attribute everything that has happened to the self. Thus, it is not surprising that the child cognitively processes the abuse as having been caused by someone and the self is blamed since she was less powerful. The following questions are comments made by adult clients of the author that reflect the confusion, cause and effect and egocentric thinking that is typical of a child: Why did someone who said they loved me hurt me? Why did not my mother or some other adult protect and take care of me? Why did something that is wrong sometimes feel good? Since answers to these questions require a more developed level of thinking (formal operational), the child logically concludes that the incest must be her fault or that there is something wrong with the self.

Even though Piaget indicates that formal operational thinking (thinking that can hypothesize reasons outside the self that cause events to happen and understand that other people can think and behave differently than the self) only begins at age 12, such hypothetical thinking is not fully developed until adulthood and continues to develop throughout the life span given healthy conditions and experiences. But, suffering a childhood trauma such as sexual abuse creates a bio-psycho-social disorder (Trotter & Gorski, 1991) with the consequence that development is interrupted and often remains at the level when the abuse began. As a result, the misconception of self-cause and guilt is carried into adulthood as well as the concrete operational thinking that blames the self and other issues surrounding the abuse.

The client remembers herself as having had more power and control over decisions as a child than what actually was possible. The adult survivor often forgets the basic characteristics of children, and needs to be reminded and helped to discover those childlike characteristics that were buried with the loss of childhood. Such child characteristics are trusting and faithful, curious with a sense of wondering, honest and open with feelings, creative, resilient, loving, flexible, forgiving and mourn easily, courageous with optimism, friendly, laugh often, relaxed, sensitive, unhurried, like to move and play and vulnerable until taught otherwise (Benson & Stewart, 1979; Coles, 1967-77; Welter, 1984). Interestingly, that the characteristics of a child are also the characteristics of a fully functioning person (Rogers, 1963). The counselor when working with a survivor is helping to enhance the characteristics that the child once had but lies buried beneath the hurt of abuse and nonacceptance. The adult survivor has forgotten how vulnerable and trusting she was when the incest began and that compliance was easily secured by the perpetrator (Bass & Davis, 1988; Engel, 1982; Hayes, 1990). Other developmental areas of the survivor's life were also altered when the exposure to physical, sexual or emotional abuse occurred. Thus, the counselor needs to listen intently for all aspects of the client so that the client feels free to grow as a whole person not just as a survivor.

By spending time with children, the survivor can return to the activities of being a child where development was left and begin to reclaim lost childlike qualities. Spending time with a person of another generation becomes a healing, genuine and caring intervention that respects the dignity of all those involved and draws upon the inherent helping qualities of people.

Counseling Process

New growth cannot occur until healing has begun. Healing occurs through forgiveness and an atmosphere of acceptance and empathy. Counseling must address not only emotions but cognition as well. Control of what is discussed must always be in the hands of the client (Chu, 1992). It is only through total acceptance and identification of feelings and attitudes that emerge in the process that the client is empowered (Rogers, 1980).

As counseling continues, the process of forgiving the perpetrator often occurs before the survivor forgives the self (Fitzgibbons, 1986). As Rogers (1969) said, "Much significant learning is acquired through doing" (p. 162). Thus, the forgiving process is not only a change in affect but must also include changes in the behavioral and cognitive realms. Intergenerational connections can be the behavioral component of helping the client to let go of self-blame, come to self-forgiveness and begin to emotionally/socially develop again. Intergenerational relationships provide qualities that are not found within a peer relationship, such as less competition, interdependency, less need for approval, enrichment through differences, mentoring, teaching, connections to the past and the future, an outlet for emotional needs, heightened awareness of life processes and less defensiveness (Benson & Stewart, 1979; Welter, 1984). Chu (1992) indicated that the development of a support network outside the counseling relationship is very important to prevent dependence upon the counselor. More importantly, developing relationships outside the counseling relationship teaches social and coping skills and help the client empower herself.

Relationship with a Child

The purpose of encouraging a relationship with a child is to help the client view the world through the child's eyes in order to discover the child's thinking and feeling process and how the client may have felt and responded as a child. The forming of a relationship with a child by the client can be done in a variety of ways. At the forefront of any intervention should be the ethical concerns of the client using a relationship with a child for her own benefit. The author has also found it very important to ethically address why a survivor might abuse someone else, i.e. act out his/her own powerlessness by having power over someone else. It is important that the survivor respect and discover the healthy aspects of another person and not just the power one can have over another.

After the aforementioned issues have been addressed, the client is asked to begin observing children. This observation may occur in the home, schools, stores, church and other such places that the client frequents. It is helpful for the client to observe children of all ages but it is particularly important to observe children of the age when the client was victimized. The client is asked to journal or to remember what activities were observed, what comments were said between children during the activities, how conflicts were resolved and how each child might be viewing his/her world at any particular time. The journal or observations are processed in the counseling session with the counselor attending to details that are the same as the client has felt, experienced and talked about during sessions. Due to family-of-origin dynamics (Titelman, 1987), the client will select significant observations that will parallel her own past experiences (these experiences have meaning to her). Through the observations, the client will begin to discover that conflict occurs often and the child with less power will compromise or give in to others in order to maintain the relationship. Likewise, the client may have agreed to the sexual activities to maintain the relationship or because she did not have the power to change the conditions.

Another intergenerational intervention is to discover the activities that the client liked to do as a child and then find opportunities to do those activities with other children. Organizations such as community recreation, camps, 4-H, scouting, big friends programs, teaching at church and aiding in schools provide opportunities for adults to become more involved with children. The client needs to be encouraged to play or do activities with children. Relationships are most often begun by doing tasks or activities with others. Most relationships other than counseling do not begin by just talking; it is an activity or purpose that brings people together that begins the communication process. Therefore, the client is asked to meet at least three to five times with children so that familiarity can develop.

The client will naturally begin to form a closer relationship with one or two children. A friendship with a child of the same age as when the client was victimized can provide the trust for the client to ask significant questions. These questions can be developed from the client's own concerns. Through talking with the child or children, the client naturally begins to discover how trusting children are with adults. Through self-reflection, the client can begin to analyze her own particular family dynamics and conclude why the abuse was not disclosed or addressed and why she might have sought out the perpetrator for attention and love that was lacking. This can be a very painful process as the client gains new information and begins to allow the self to feel as a child again. The counselor must constantly reflect the feelings and empathize with the pain. As the anger and revenge surface, the client may want to confront the perpetrator. However, it is important for more healing of the self to occur. The anger that was previously directed at the self and caused the depression surfaces and often is transferred to the perpetrator and the family. Until the client feels empowered and in control of the self by the discovery of her unique identity, the client is not ready to confront the perpetrator. A great majority of premature confrontations with the perpetrator result in the client being emotionally and verbally abused again by denial and rejection (Engel, 1989). The motivation for a confrontation is to let the perpetrator know that the secret of incest no longer has power over her and how she has changed as a result of growing beyond her past.

To gain this new sense of self, the survivor is encouraged to continue relationships with children. Again, the survivor is encouraged to do activities with them. In the process of playing and physical activity, the survivor will reconnect with the child within (Abrams, 1990). In the reconnecting process, many memories may resurface. The memories will frequently need to be processed in the counseling sessions. During the reconnecting process, the counselor continues to use outside relationships as a learning intervention resource with the client. The following is a case sample from the author's counseling practice that describes the use of intergenerational resources.

Lisa came to marital counseling with her husband concerning issues of infertility. Within the first session, issues of sexuality surfaced as I attempted to listen and identify feelings and attitudes that seemed to prevent the couple from coming closer at this time of crisis. After hearing many of the characteristics of incest, I gently inquired about possible abuse from her older brother. She began crying and asked to have counseling time alone. In the course of the next two sessions, feelings of guilt and self-blame continued to surface. As a result, I suggested that she might appreciate getting to know what she was like at the age that the incest had begun, eight years old. She readily agreed and decided that a friend's niece from a single parent home would probably enjoy more time with her. She had previously babysat for her. Within two activity visits, Lisa discovered the types of fast food places and activities that the child liked. Lisa then asked the child to go to a fast food place that was not one of the child's favorites on the next visit. Lisa discovered how easy it was to talk a child into doing something that the child does not want to do because the child values the relationship. Lisa was encouraged to be honest and pick a place she preferred although it was not necessary to actually eat there with her friend. Lisa also discovered new joy in doing child activities such as swinging, playing dolls, coloring and watching cartoons. These were only a few of the benefits of the relationship. As a result, Lisa began to see that the abuse was not her fault and the forgiveness and guilt began to dissipate as she grew into a new sense of knowing about herself not only as an adult but also as a child.

An Adult Relationship

Another intervention using intergenerational resources is to help the client connect with an older adult. Often a characteristic that emerges in the counseling process is unexplainable anger toward the mother. The client is angry on an unconscious level at the mother for not protecting and taking care of her when she was a child.

By encouraging the client to form relationships with older adults particularly a women, the client can begin to discover what challenges are confronted in parenting and perceptions of persons of another generation. The community can provide the opportunities for the client to become involved in activities that the client enjoys while being with older persons. Such organizations and programs as senior citizens, recreation centers, nursing homes, churches, social services and hospital groups welcome persons becoming involved in their activities. Again, the client needs to participate in the activities at least three to five times and the counselor needs to warn the client that she probably won't feel comfortable with the group at first. Relationships and communication about significant topics most often develop around a common interest or activity and occur over time.

The client is again invited to ask questions concerning parenting, the disappointments and joys of living and other issues that pertain to the client.

Relationships with older persons can help the client look to the future as well. The older adult can become a mentor and friend that is more unconditionally accepting of the client than the family is and can teach parenting skills that the client did not experience within a dysfunctional family. Social skills in meeting and talking with others on a trusting, intimate level often occurs more easily with older adult friends. An accepting, trusting friendship with an older person provides the healing, growth-producing environment for the client to begin trusting self and others again. The potential of any intergenerational friendship can be the healing catalyst for many unfinished issues. But when abuse has occurred, such a friendship can even provide more support and growth for the issues of the incest survivor.

Conclusion

Due to a mobile and changing American society, intergenerational support systems that were once a frequent part of the American family are no longer universally present. Encouraging intergenerational relationships can be a counseling intervention that enhances the client's growth and development. Counseling is only effective when the client is able to transfer the skills and understandings learned during sessions to the everyday world. Developing healthy friendships with others outside the family can provide growth that cannot be found within the incestuous family. For the incest survivor, intergenerational relationships become the connection to the past for healing and the connection to the future for hope. The challenge for the person-centered counselor is to seek out and utilize meaningful, caring, warm and unconditional acceptance for clients that can be found in inter-generational relationships.

Marlene M. Kuskie, Ed.D. is with the Department of Counseling and School Psychology, the University of Nebraska at Kearney.

References

Abrams, J. (1990). **Reclaiming the inner child.** Los Angeles, CA: Jeremy P. Tarcher, Inc.

Bass, E. & Davis, L. (1988). **The courage to heal.** New York: Harper & Row.

Benson, D. & Stewart, S. (1979). **The ministry of the child.** Nashville: Abingdon.

Bessett, L. (1985). **Child victims: Evaluating, understanding and treating sexually abused children.** Paper presented at meeting of National Association of Social Workers, Washington, D.C.

Chu, J. (1992). The therapeutic roller coaster: Dilemmas in the treatment of childhood abuse survivors. **Journal of Psychotherapy Practice and Research, 1,** 351-370.

Coles, R. (1967-77). **Children of crisis.** Boston: Little, Brown and Co.

Courtois, C. (1988). **Healing the incest wound.** New York: W. W. Norton & Company.

Courtois, D. & Sprei, J. (1988). Retrospective incest therapy for women. In L. E. Walker (Ed.). **Handbook of sexual abuse of children.** New York: Springer.

Courtois, D. & Watts, D. (1982). Counseling adult women who experienced incest in childhood or adolescence. **Personnel and Guidance Journal,** 275-279.

Engel, B. (1982). **The right to innocence.** Los Angeles: Jeremy P. Tarcher.

Faria, G. & Belohlavek, M. (1984). Treating female adult survivors of childhood incest. **Social Casework,** 465-471.

Finkelhor, D. (1984). **Child sexual abuse: New theory and research.** New York: The Free Press.

Finkelhor, D. & Browne, A. (1985). The traumatic impact of child sexual abuse: A conceptualization. **American Journal of Orthopsychiatry, 55,** 530-541.

Fitzgibbons, T. (1986). The cognitive and emotive uses of forgiveness in the treatment of anger. **Psychotherapy, 23**, 629-633.

Gelinas, D. (1983). The persisting negative effects of incest. **Psychiatry, 46**, 312-332.

Hayes, L. (1988). Incest: A violation of trust. **Guideposts, 30**, 1-3.

Herman, J. (1981). **Father-daughter incest.** Cambridge, MA: Harvard University Press.

Hoagwood, K. & Stewart, J. (1989). Sexually abused children's perceptions of family functioning. **Child and Adolescent Social Work, 6**, 139-149.

Janoff-Bulman, R. (1979). Characterological versus behavioral self-blame: Inquiries into depression and rape. **Journal of Personality and Social Psychology, 37**, 1798-1809.

Janoff-Bulman, R. & Frieze, I. (1983). A theoretical perspective for understanding reactions to victimization. **Journal of Social Issues, 39**, 1-18.

Jehu, D., Gazan, M. & Klassen, C. (1985). Common therapeutic targets among women who were sexually abused in childhood. **Feminist perspectives on social work and human sexuality**, 25-45.

Joy, S. (1987). Retrospective presentations of incest: Treatment strategies for use with adult women. **Journal of Counseling and Development, 65**, 317-319.

Kirschenbaum, H. (1979). **On becoming Carl Rogers.** New York: Dell Publishing.

Mayer, A. (1983). **Incest: A treatment manual for therapy with victims, spouses and offenders.** Holmes Beach, FL: Learning Publications.

Meiselman, K. (1978). **Incest: A psychological study of cause and effects with treatment recommendations.** San Francisco: Jossey-Bass.

Miller, D. & Porter, C. (1983). Self-blame in victims of violence. **Journal of Social Issues, 39**, 139-152.

Mrazek, P. & Bentovim, A. (1981). Incest and the dysfunctional family system. In P.

Mrazek & C. Kempe (Eds.) **Sexually abused children and their families.** New York: Pergamon Press.

Piaget, J. & Inhelder, B. (1969). **Psychology of the child.** New York: Basic Books.

Poston, C. & Lison, K. (1989). **Reclaiming our lives.** Boston: Little, Brown and Company.

Rogers, C. (1963). The concept of the fully functioning person. **Psychotherapy: Theory, Research, and Practice, 1,** 17-26.

Rogers, C. (1969). **Freedom to learn.** Columbus, OH: Charles E. Merrill Publishing.

Rogers, C. (1978). The formative tendency. **Journal of Humanistic Psychology, 18,** 23-26.

Rogers, C. (1980). **A way of being.** Boston: Houghton Mifflin.

Rosenfeld, A., Nadelson, C., Krieger, M. & Backman, J. (1979). Incest and sexual abuse of children. **Journal of American Academy of Child Psychiatry, 16,** 327-39.

Russell, D. (1986). **The secret trauma: Incest in the lives of girls and women.** New York: Basic Books.

Saunders, B., Murphy, S., & McClure, S. (1987). **Assessment of family structure variables of cases in intra-familial child sexual abuse.** Paper presented at American Orthopsychiatry Association.

Summit, R. (1983). The child sexual abuse syndrome. **Child abuse and neglect, 7,** 177-193.

Summit, R. & Kryso, J. (1978). Sexual abuse of children: A clinical spectrum. **American Journal of Orthopsychiatry, 48,** 237-251.

Titelman, P. (1987). **The therapist's own family.** Northvale, NJ: Jason Aronson.

Trotter, C. & Gorski, T. (1991). Relapse and the survivors of childhood abuse. **FOCUS,** (February-March), 30-39.

Welter, P. (1984). **Learning from children.** Wheaton, IL: Tyndale.

An Exploration on the themes of Congruence, Incongruence and Alcohol Use

Richard Bryant-Jefferies

I work for a community drug and alcohol service in the UK. My role has been that of alcohol counsellor with a specific remit to work in Primary Health Care. The counselling approach that I work with is client-centred. Working in this way within the field of alcohol counselling I have been struck by the issue of congruence and incongruence both in the client and the therapist as an agent of change, or as a block to change. It has led me to reflect on what congruence actually means in terms of the experiencing of the client who is using alcohol either out of habit or as a means of coping with psychological discomfort. I have been left wondering about how alcohol, as it affects the nervous system, can interrupt congruent experiencing. It has left me, too, with a conviction that the congruence of the therapist is a vitally important contributing factor in encouraging alcohol-affected clients to seek their own congruence, and that incongruence in the therapist will very likely block growthful movement in the client.

Rogers (1990) himself wrote:

> The more the therapist is himself or herself in the relationship, putting up no professional front or personal facade, the greater is the likelihood that the client will change and grow in a constructive manner. Genuineness means that the therapist is openly

being the feelings and attitudes that are flowing within at the moment. There is a close matching, or congruence, between what is being experienced at the gut level, what is present in awareness, and what is expressed to the client. (p. 135)

This presents us with a clear view of the challenge of congruence for the therapist. Working with clients for whom there can be a lot of denial and a pattern of secrecy present, congruence in the therapist is crucially important if it is also to be encouraged within the client.

Trusting the client

A dilemma that I, and I believe most alcohol workers, face, is whether to work with the alcohol problem that the person is presenting, or whether to focus on the underlying difficulties that are being dealt with through the use of alcohol.

I would suggest that the person who knows best is the client. It is my belief that they will be genuinely encouraged to focus on the area that is of greatest urgency to them by the presence of congruence in the therapist. My willingness to be real and to maintain as much as I can a realistic perspective and open engagement with my experiencing will enable the client to achieve the same. In doing so, they may well find themselves having to choose to face up to incongruencies. My sense is that, as the client risks greater congruence within the therapeutic relationship and finds it is both acceptable within that relationship and deeply satisfying to them, they will move towards a clearer recognition of the presence of incongruence. Blocks to the accurate experiencing and communicating of what is present within them will be lifted or removed, perhaps dissolved might be a better word, enabling greater transparency to emerge.

This perspective is, I believe, extremely challenging for many who work in the field of alcohol misuse. I have encountered frequently attitudes that break down into:

- The client cannot be trusted

- The client does not know what is good for him or her
- The client has to reach rock bottom before they can change
- The client does not have his/her own inner resources to make changes

I challenge these and certainly PCA challenges them. Rogers indicated his strong belief that:

"the basic nature of the human being, when functioning freely, is constructive and trustworthy" (Rogers, 1961, p. 194).

I believe this is so. Clients do know what is best for them but they may need to be helped through the chemical barrier to engage with that awareness. I am convinced that if a truly facilitative environment can be created then individuals can change in constructive and fulfilling ways. This was certainly Rogers' view: "Individuals have within themselves vast resources for self-understanding and for altering their self-concepts, basic attitudes, and self-directed behaviour; these resources can be tapped if a definable climate of facilitative psychological attitudes can be provided" (Rogers, 1980, p. 115).

The problem that often arises is whether that environment can be maintained over a significant enough length of time so that change can be sustainable. Is my alcohol-dependent client going to change significantly in their outlook and self-concept through 1 hour's therapy a week? Maybe, maybe not. It may not stop them drinking, but it may begin to move their self-concept away from whatever is sustaining their need to drink. It may help them begin to experience a greater free flow of congruent awareness such that they recognise for themselves their need for change. It may enable them to own a desire to move on from where they currently are. However, sustainable change may well need more frequent contact initially to help the person really to begin to experience other possibilities within themselves, to experience being in an empathic and non-judgmental relationship, to touch the exquisite edge of authenticity and to realise that they experience a sense of self that, whilst it may not always be comfortable, is more compelling.

They are then faced with some significant choices. Authenticity in the relationship brings the person more out into the open and as he or she begins to move towards becoming themselves and more open to their personal experiencing. "He realises that he can choose to continue to hide behind a facade, or that he can take the risks involved in being himself; that he is free agent who has it within his power to destroy another, or himself, and also the power to enhance himself and others" (Rogers, 1961, p. 203). Rogers goes on to suggest that: "Faced with this naked reality of decision, he chooses to move in the direction of being himself" (p. 203).

It is not that the person's problems go away; they remain and yet fresh possibilities may also be glimpsed. It is, however, also possible that the person faced with insurmountable difficulties may choose further self-harm or even suicide. It happens. People can drink themselves into a suicidal frame of mind. I believe that I have a responsibility out of my respect for the person I am working with to express any feelings I may have if I am aware of this possibility. Whilst the presence of empathy, congruence, psychological contact and unconditional positive regard can be sufficient to move a person towards positive, growth-enhancing choices, I also recognise that a heavy drinking session could move a person into a suicidal state of mind—almost two-thirds of suicide attempts in the UK are linked to heavy drinking (Department of Health, 1993).

I am constantly left with the question: Can I trust my client? Rogers suggested that

"It is the client who knows what hurts, what directions to go, what problems are crucial. It began to occur to me that unless I had a need to demonstrate my own cleverness and learning, I would do better to rely upon the client for the direction of movement in the process" (Rogers, 1961, pp. 11-12).

What am I trusting them to do? To behave in a particular way? My trust has to be that they will make the choices that are right for them. I believe that this will occur. However, I do have a concern as to whether the seriously alcohol-affected client is able to do this. They may well be experiencing encouragement from the effects of the alcohol to pursue a self-destruct course of action. Is this a freely chosen action, or does it stem from the effects of the alcohol on the nervous system? I have worked with too many people whose behaviours change under heavy alcohol use: it may be hurt and anger from past abuse, but it may be chemically triggered.

I am left asking myself, can I trust my client under the influence of heavy alcohol intake to choose a constructive direction in their life? The crucial part of Rogers' comment quoted earlier: "the basic nature of the human being, when functioning freely, is constructive and trustworthy" (Rogers, 1961, p. 194) is the factor of "functioning freely." Is the alcohol-affected client, or any other chemically-affected client, able to truly function freely? I can trust their person, but I may not be able to trust their behaviour to take a constructive direction. I believe this is an authentic perspective and if I was to feel this strongly with a client I would expect to hear myself voice it. Such congruence on my part may touch the client deeply and, because it is an expression of genuine concern, it is much more likely to make an impression than a judgemental response that is full of an "I know best" attitude. There are those who will consider the person with the alcohol problem as inferior and incapable of change, that they have a disease and need to be 'treated'. Their unique personhood and rich potential is ignored and diminished through this attitude.

I am challenged to trust my client's choices, and for my trust to be real it has to be rooted in my own congruent experiencing. Where there is no congruence in the therapist then the trust will, in my view, be irresponsible and the relationship will not be authentic. We will end up with an "anything goes" situation which is not PCA and I, as the therapist, will lose my credibility. I may be experiencing that which the alcohol is blocking them from experiencing and it becomes vital that I voice what is present for me which may be concern, or it may be to offer a perspective that is present for me, or a sense of the rightness of a choice that the client is making. The classic example is the client who is a dependent drinker, getting through a bottle of spirits a day: he tells you he stopped yesterday; he is shaking and really struggling to keep any kind of conscious focus in his relationship with you, he may even be hallucinating. You could sit there conveying a pseudo-trust that all is well, but authenticity calls for you to express any concerns you may have as it is quite possible that your client is in a life-threatening condition from alcohol withdrawal. The PCA will require you to respond to the client's inner world of experience and your congruent flow of experiencing. Your respect for the client will demand of you action in seeking a medical intervention.

Rock bottom

Does the heavy drinker need to hit rock bottom in order to change? Who defines rock-bottom? There is a culture that seems to define it as "lose everything". Not everyone needs to reach this low point and many clients can recognise that they have to make changes long before everything is lost. But there is often a need for a trigger. It could be that someone close to them dies of an alcohol-related condition, or that they experience a drink-driving offence. It could be pain and discomfort that they are experiencing from their own alcohol use. It will vary from person to person. What the client needs in that moment is a facilitative environment in which they can be supported in engaging with what is present within themselves. Many reach rock-bottom because this facilitative environment has not been offered. Often it is believed that it has been, but my view is that it is usually very conditional and judgmental. Having said that, sadly it is a fact that there will also be those people who do lose everything.

Alcohol effects

When working with clients who are using alcohol as a psychological prop, the importance of congruence needs to be emphasised if the therapeutic relationship is to be constructive, and the client is to move towards greater congruence and self-reliance as a person in their own individual and unique right. Through the therapeutic process the client develops an "increasing openness to experience" (Rogers, 1961, p. 187). The impressions that impact upon him or her are experienced with reduced distortion. However, I believe that alcohol is a factor that can, and does, reduce this. Rogers (1961) writes that: "If a person could be fully open to his experience, however, every stimulus—whether originating within the organism or in the environment—would be freely relayed through the nervous system without being distorted by any defensive mechanism" (pp. 187-188).

Yet it is not only defences that affect the functioning of the nervous system. We know that alcohol suppresses the nervous system, interfering with the free relay of the stimulus. It is hard enough when we have psychological blocks hindering free flow, but when chemical suppressants such as alcohol are introduced into the body's biological make-up, further difficulties are going to be created for the person who is seeking to grow towards greater congruence. Alcohol blurs our awareness and can cause us to misinterpret situations and impressions. The classic example of this is the person who looks across the bar at someone who has a level of alcohol in their body that is affecting their accurate understanding of impression. It is seen as a threat; "What're you starin' at then mate?" leading to a possibly volatile situation with verbal or physical assault a possibility.

Also, alcohol initially reduces our inhibitions, freeing us up to behave in ways that are not normally our 'style'. For some this will be the great attraction of alcohol, particularly when they need to face a situation that for them is experienced as difficult: perhaps a social situation, or a tense relational problem. Is the alcohol enabling them to be more themselves and therefore more congruent, or is it enabling them to be something other than themselves and therefore less congruent? Or can we say that it doesn't matter, how they are is how they are regardless of whether alcohol is involved or not, and, if they are congruent to the chemically affected experiencing, then they are truly congruent? I believe this is a question that must be addressed in a period of history when we are more chemically affected than at any other time in terms of alcohol and drug use, chemicals in foods and substances we make contact with, and pollution in the air and the water. I am left wondering whether chemically affected congruence is true congruence, or a kind of false congruence.

Now, in terms of alcohol, inhibition goes first, then co-ordination is affected. The more we drink, the greater the effect. With altered co-ordination comes altered communication. Reduced inhibition may have left the person communicating more than they might normally do, which means they may find greater congruency in their words, but as co-ordination is affected then they may find it increasingly difficult to think clearly and to engage the words that accurately reflect the experiencing. So we might conclude that, whilst initially alcohol might enhance congruence, continued use becomes a block to the ability to be congruent. Having said that, the fact that alcohol reduces inhibitions means as well that the person who is drinking is only being true to chemically-affected organismic functioning.

Incongruencies can develop when a person's self-concept is felt to be under threat. Anxiety develops and a process of defence occurs seeking to obstruct the free and accurate experiencing of the threat. So consider the alcohol-using client (1) with a negative self-concept who experiences warmth, genuineness, empathy from a therapist that sends the message to them that they are OK, they are valued, they are worthy of being prized. This is, for them, a direct assault on their self-concept. How might they counter this? One way will be to stop seeing the therapist. Another way will be to increase the alcohol intake. The latter is a challenge to the client-centred alcohol counsellor. Can they accept that their way of working may induce in the client a choice to take more alcohol? The effect will be to exacerbate the client's incongruence. So, for the drinking client who is using alcohol to either deal with the discomfort of a poor self-image, or to deal with the experiencing that fosters their poor self-image, things may well get worse before they get better.

However, other drinking clients with no underlying emotional need to take alcohol will have developed a view of themselves as a heavy drinker (2)—this will be their identity in terms of their own experiencing and may have become well established over a period of time. It will be a part of their self-concept. They may struggle to change this as their experience continues to match their self-concept. Congruency is present. Their alcohol use is rooted in congruence.

What I think this suggests is that alcohol use may be rooted in incongruence for some and congruence for others, depending on their history and the meanings they have internalised into their self-concept.

In (2) above, damage from the alcohol use may well be making an impact on them, and within the organism there may be signals urging change by means of physical discomfort or even pain. So it is a form of 'false congruence' because, whilst their experience matches their self-concept and they communicate this, their organism may be experiencing damage which is not being consciously acknowledged. Therefore incongruence has to be present within the functioning of the whole person.

Let us look a little more closely at the person who is drinking to cope with low self-worth.

Stage 1

The person turns to alcohol to cope, finding they are unable to bear the feelings or thoughts they have towards themselves. A distorted self-concept has been generated through negative and unrealistic conditioning, leaving them with a sense of being inadequate and useless. Incongruence is present. "I'm just no good as a human being. The only thing that relieves my anguish is having a few glasses of brandy in the evening."

Stage 2

Alcohol anaesthetises the discomfort, the person is no longer in touch with the flow of uncomfortable experiencing passing through them. Incongruence is present. "I'm OK, really, I never think much about the accident now. How much do I drink? Oh, about a half a bottle of scotch a day. I feel really good on it."

Stage 3

A significant life event occurs that causes a breakthrough of congruence towards the flow of experiencing. They are, if you like, jolted out of the anaesthetic. They experience their reality as they see themselves, including feelings towards themselves, as an alcohol-dependent person. The break-through fuels an urge to be congruent, to be real to themselves recognising that there is a strength in this. However, this is set against the nagging urge that remains to blot out the difficult feelings, the urge to anaesthetise, the established habit. "What am I doing to myself? I would never have had that accident if I hadn't been drinking. I haven't had a drink since. I still feel a craving to, particularly when I am on my own, but I really don't want to go back to how it was."

At this point, two directions are possible.

Stage 4a

The anaesthetic (alcohol) is chosen. The security of familiar incongru-ence is returned to.

Stage 4b

There is a definite attempt made to hold on to the flow of experiencing and to cut out the anaesthetic (alcohol) so that the experiencing may be genuine. Greater congruence is achieved.

I would like to suggest that congruence is linked to the relationship between the organism, awareness and communication. When we are affected as an organism by something, we are aware of the impact and we experience and interpret it accurately; we are able to communicate the experience in a manner that matches what is happening, we are congruent. There are no blocks in the flow. So let us consider the following:

a) A person who is organismically in pain from alcohol intake—actual physical damage may exist, or it could be discomfort present in feelings or thoughts. "I know I've got liver damage and my stomach's not too good. It can be really painful some days. I want to be healthy and get my life together again. I really want alcohol out of my life."

He or she is conscious of this damage and the reason why. They accept this.

He or she is able to communicate freely their pain/discomfort, where it stems from, and their need to be pain free. This person is ready to address the issue of their alcohol intake. They are congruent.

b) A person who is organismically in pain from alcohol intake—actual physical damage may exist, or it could be discomfort present in feelings or thoughts. "I really don't like the anxiety attacks I'm getting some days around late morning. I never used to be that anxious. I want to find a way of stopping it, there must be some kind of psychological exercise I can do? The only thing that eases the anxiety is to have a drink. That seems to be one good solution, it certainly isn't part of the problem." (Anxiety attacks and withdrawal symptoms can be easily confused!)

He or she denies the link between drinking and the damage

He or she communicates their desire to be pain free

This person is unlikely to maintain abstention from alcohol. There is incongruence.

c) A person who is organismically in pain from alcohol intake—actual physical damage may exist, or it could be discomfort present in feelings or thoughts. "I thought I'd come to see you. I'm getting pain in my stomach and my memory doesn't seem too sharp these days. I feel so tired and listless. I've been to the doctor for tablets to pick me up. He suggested I come and talk to you." (Thinks: It's the alcohol, I know it is, but I feel so ashamed and I don't want anyone to know. What am I going to do?)

He or she is aware that alcohol is the cause and accepts this.

He or she is unable to communicate their need for help for fear of the alcohol problem becoming known. There is incongruence. It is going to be difficult for this person to change.

Organism, awareness and communication

Reflecting on this led me to think about the relationship between the organism, awareness and communication and I now see this in the form of a triangle:

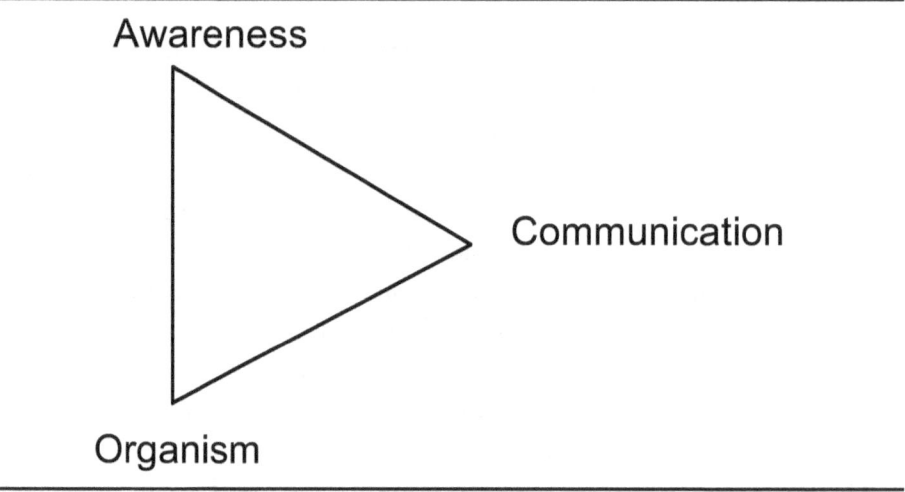

Figure 1

When congruence is present we have a free flow between the points of the triangle (Figure 1). What is present within the organism is accurately experienced in awareness and can be openly communicated to others.

Bearing this limitation in mind, let us still consider how it might represent congruence and incongruence in relation to the client who is drinking excessively. What I would like to suggest is that we can have a congruent relationship between two aspects of the triangle yet incongruence elsewhere. Consider the following: in each the discomfort is related to alcohol use, creating physical damage in the individual:

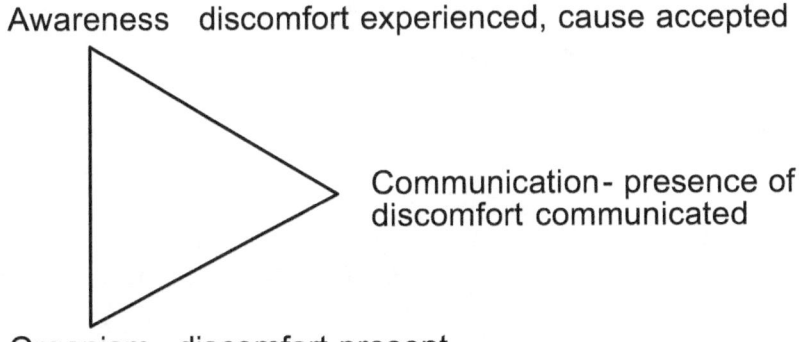

Awareness discomfort experienced, cause accepted

Communication- presence of
discomfort communicated

Organism- discomfort present

Figure 2

In Figure 2 there is a clear and open response to the experienced effects of alcohol use. It could be summed up in the words: "I'm feeling bad. I know why and what it's doing to me. I can feel it. The drinking is causing me problems. I have to do something about it. I want to break this habit." The thinking and experiencing process behind the words will be the same. In this situation I would argue that the client is experiencing a state of congruence towards their drinking. Everything matches up, there is a minimum of distortion. There is power in this experience and I have found when working with clients who bring this congruence into a session there is real hope of lasting change. My own congruence will remain important as well: they are being real with themselves and with me; that the last thing they need is for me to undermine this by what I bring into the relationship.

However, we can represent other situations by using solid lines for a free flow between points, and dotted lines where the flow is distorted or blocked. The following are examples:

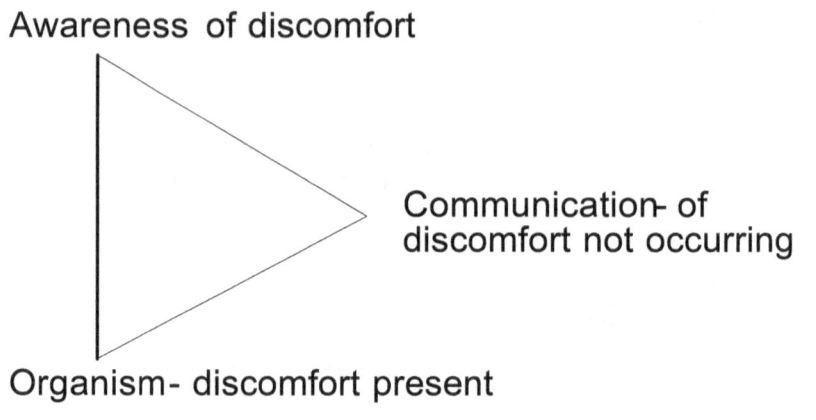

Awareness of discomfort

Communication of discomfort not occurring

Organism- discomfort present

Figure 3

Here (Figure 3) there is a flow between what is present within the organism and awareness. However it is not being communicated. There is incongruence. "I'm OK." (*Thinks*: I'm not telling you about my discomfort, I don't want anyone to know about my drinking).

Awareness of discomfort not present

Discomfort not communicatec

Organism- discomfort present

Figure 4

In the above (Figure 4) whilst discomfort exists within the organism, this is not being registered in the individual's awareness or being communicated verbally or through behaviour. Again, there exists within the person a state of incongruence. "I'm OK, I really am." (*Thinks*: I really am OK, never felt better.)

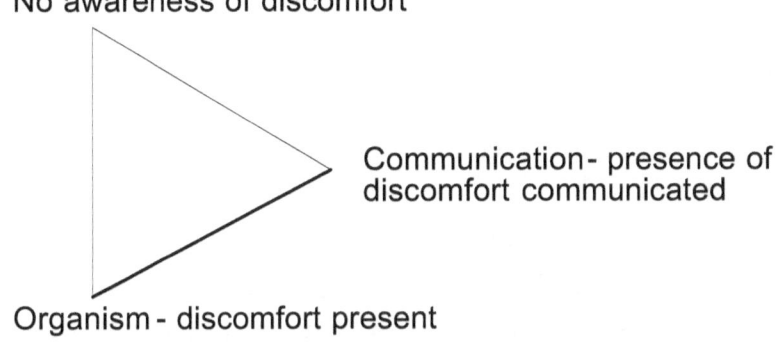

No awareness of discomfort

Communication- presence of discomfort communicated

Organism - discomfort present

Figure 5

In this triangle (Figure 5) the discomfort experienced within the organism is present and communicated, perhaps through adaptive behaviour: however the individual is unaware that it is happening. Once more, incongruence is present in the person. "It's good to be here and everything feels fine. Sorry I didn't make it last week, these things happen when you're leading a busy life you know." (Alcohol use can impair memory function. It is being communicated to the counsellor, but is not something the client is really aware of.)

Let us define some of the situations in which drinking may be incongruent or congruent.

Incongruent alcohol use:

- anaesthetic effect to maintain an avoidance of discomforting feelings, emotions or thoughts that are present within the person.
- when alcohol-related physical damage is occurring and recognised but it is denied to others;
- physical damage is occurring but has not been experienced and no link has been made to alcohol use;
 Congruent alcohol use:
- there is a fit between the drinking behaviour and the person's self-concept;
- there is an intention to reduce organismic discomfort that is experienced;
- physical damage is occurring, experienced and communicated but the link with alcohol use is not recognised.

Where does this leave us? Perhaps we need to think in phases. Is there an incongruent phase and a congruent phase? Do clients move from one to the other? The habitual drinker with no discomfort and no underlying emotional issues fuelling drinking behaviour is congruent in terms of drinking. When discomfort arises then incongruence may develop, it will depend on how the person responds. If they deny it to themselves or to others then incongruence emerges and the likelihood of change is less than if they are open to it, accept its cause and are able to communicate it to others. The latter will be a congruent state. Therefore congruence towards a simply habitual drinking behaviour could be seen as the most likely condition for change to occur.

I think this needs to be dwelt on a little more. Rogers suggests that incongruence in the client is a core condition for constructive personality change to occur, that "the client, is in a state of incongruence, being vulnerable or anxious" (Rogers, 1990, p. 221). This may be so towards underlying emotional difficulties and distortions in self-concept, which I believe

Rogers was referring to, but with regard to alcohol use it is possible that it is the congruence of the client that can become the necessary factor in promoting an urge within them to pursue a path of personality change. It is the power of experiencing alcohol-related harm, knowing that it is alcohol, knowing that they no longer wish to experience this and actively voicing this need that indicates a readiness for change.

I can simplistically differentiate clients into those who expect the counsellor to have a magic wand and to solve their problem for them, and those who own the problem and are themselves seeking direction as to what *they* can do for the best. There is something about the ownership of an habitual drinking problem that is linked to the presence of congruence. To not own it when you are aware of it as a fact in your experience and to not own that you are the agent of change in your life, I would argue, is to be incongruent and to undermine the possibility of change.

Yet there is also a congruence in a client's genuine feeling of helplessness in the face of a habit that they feel unable to break free of. It may well be real and without medical intervention there may be no break away from dependent drinking. In this case, their congruence may be such that they are overwhelmed by helplessness and simply not seek help or support. When they do, the valuing and prizing of the person behind the alcohol use will be crucial, along with the congruence of the therapist who will be entering into this helpless world as a companion and, perhaps, offering a source of strength by their presence to help the client begin to believe that change is possible.

However, when there are underlying emotional issues that the alcohol has been used to cope with to a point of becoming habitual, then, until the feelings are engaged with, understood and experienced accurately by the drinker, there is less likelihood of sustainable change, whatever the intervention. Incongruence will be present. The urge for change may then be triggered by the discomfort of the incongruence with respect to the feelings that underlie the drinking, or congruence towards the drinking given a clear recognition and ownership of the fact that it is making things worse.

We might also have to bear in mind that congruent use of alcohol can generate incongruence as well in that the transparency and free flow is lost; accurate experiencing and symbolisation is lost; organismic discomfort may not reach awareness as the alcohol affects the central nervous system.

The triangles given earlier I think illustrate the situation for habitual drinkers with no underlying emotional issues fuelling alcohol use. When this situation is present it is possible for the person to be congruent towards their actual drinking but in a state of incongruence towards their feelings. We may therefore have to consider the triangle as being multi-layered:

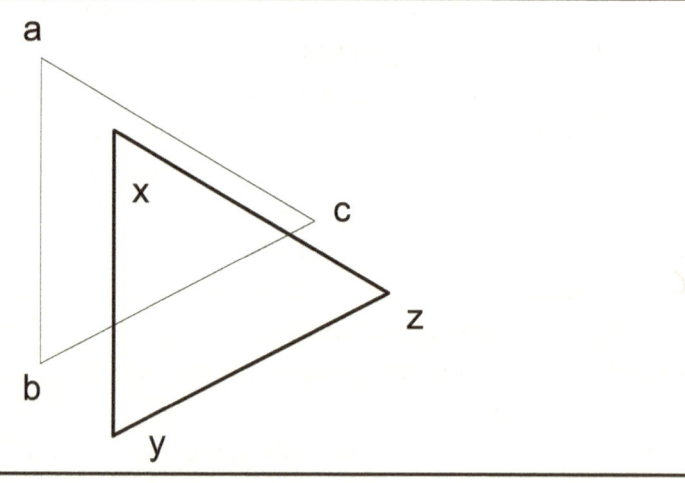

Figure 6

In this diagram (Figure 6), a-b-c reflects the incongruence when an underlying emotional trauma is unrecognised and uncommunicated, and alcohol is acting as an unintended anaesthetic. Point a represents awareness, b represents the organism or body, c represents communication, each in relation to the underlying emotional problem. The triangle x-y-z reflects congruence in so far as the physical problem of alcohol use is accurately recognised, experienced and communicated. Point x represents awareness, y represents the organism or body, z represents communication, each relating to the use of alcohol.

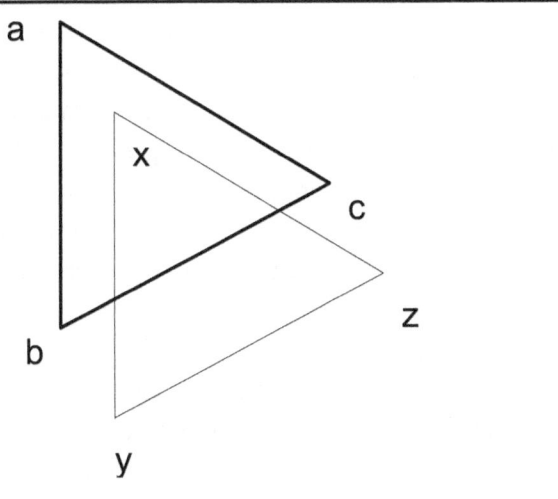

Figure 7

In Figure 7 the situation is reversed, the underlying emotional problem is recognised, experienced accurately and communicated (triangle a-b-c) however the alcohol use that has become a threat to the health of the person is not recognised or communicated (triangle x-y-z).

The situation in Figure 6 might be summed up by a client commenting: "I've got to do something about my drinking. It's making me not feel myself. I feel blurred, unable to engage with life. I know it's only a habit, I've just got to break it. It would help if I had a job and less time to have to fill."

In contrast, the situation in Figure 7 could be represented by a client saying: "I feel so empty since losing my job, I cannot seem to find fulfilment in my life. Well, the only thing that seems to satisfy me is drinking, but that's not a problem, I never get a hangover."

Conclusion

I am sure there are many other permutations to these triangles and many different triangular relationships could be formulated to try to reflect more of the whole person. I am sure we carry with us areas of our experiencing and expression that are congruent, and areas that are not. Can we ever have complete congruence across all aspects of our experience as a human being? I do not know, but I am beginning to think it unlikely, as there are so many signals passing through our central nervous system that we are not conscious of and yet which are part of our functioning as a human being. Perhaps we are not being asked to be wholly congruent as therapists, but to be congruent in the context of what is being disclosed by the client. When this is the case the potential for growth is present in the moment. Perhaps this is as much as we can hope for.

My experience of working with clients who have alcohol problems suggests to me that a large part of the difficulty lies in their sensitivity to their emotions. I believe that for some this is a cause of alcohol use, but I also believe that it can be an effect of excessive alcohol intake as well. It seems as though for some people alcohol can shut away the emotions, for others it opens them up. I feel sure this is related to congruence and incongruence in some mysterious way.

I take the view that the congruence of the therapist will enable the client to explore areas of incongruence and to seek out greater congruence within themselves. I believe this process is a trustworthy function of the therapeutic relationship. Of course, they may choose to block this by taking more alcohol. If they do not it is probably a sign that they are beginning to accept themselves as a person, making their own evaluation of themselves, and relying less on others for this. They will be more attentive to the messages that come from their organism, more able to freely interpret their meaning and make informed choices as to the action that they choose to take. However, when incongruence is present and communicated by the therapist, the client may begin to lose their own congruence, as if incongruence is unwittingly being encouraged as the norm for the relationship, or rather for the way of being within the relationship. On the other hand, the client is encouraged into greater congruence towards their world of experiencing through the presence of the therapist's congruence. This is not necessarily a conscious intention on the part of the therapist, but is a product of the client-centred way of working.

What I have sought to indicate is that conditions of congruence and incongruence are relevant factors to be considered in understanding alcohol use. There is a great deal of scope for research and discussion among those who work with this client group to produce a theory that can explain, in the context of the client-centred approach, what enables some people to be more likely to change a damaging alcohol habit than others.

Richard Bryant-Jefferies is with Acorn Community Drug and Alcohol Service, Guildford, England as an alcohol counsellor and as the co-ordinator of a Primary Health Care Alcohol Counselling Service. He also offers freelance training, counselling and supervision on alcohol issues.

References

Rogers, C. R., (1961). **On becoming a person**. London: Constable.

Rogers, C. R., (1980). **Way of being**. Boston: Houghton Mifflin.

Rogers, C. R., (1990). The therapeutic relationship. In Kirschenbaum, H, & Henderson, V. L. (Eds.), **The Carl Rogers reader**. (p. 57-152). London: Constable.

Rogers, C. R., (1990). Theory and resource. In Kirschenbaum, H, & Henderson, V. L. (Eds.), **The Carl Rogers reader**. (p. 199-257). London: Constable.

Department of Health, (1993). **Health of the nation key area handbook: mental health**. London: Her Majesty's Stationary Office.

Person-Centered Sandtray Therapy

Susan Bonner Schwarz,
& Joachim Schwarz

As therapy becomes more and more symptom centered instead of person centered it is becoming increasingly vital for humanists to speak to the emotional, relational and existential needs of individuals caught up in our psychologically disorienting times. The theories and practices of humanistic psychotherapy strive to work with the average person in search of a more meaningful life and enhanced relationship satisfaction. Serving more than a basic symptom-control function, humanistic psychology is devoted to self-actualization by developing higher levels of awareness and enhanced quality of life.

Clinical outcome research in the field point to an inability to distinguish clear differences between specific therapeutic humanistic approaches. Researchers attribute virtually all positive effects to the expectancy and general relationship factors common to all therapeutic approaches (Horvath, 1988; Prioleau, Murdick, & Brody, 1983). What actually creates change and hope in therapy is the client's motivation and the presence of a facilitating person who can offer acceptance, respect, warmth, empathy and genuineness.

That therapy is mostly a matter of revisioning hope and providing clients with a supportive, unconditional and empathetic relationship has an important implication. Keys to comprehending ourselves and each other in our meeting necessitates a continued exploration of language and nonverbal communication (Frank, 1987, 1973; Zilbergeld, 1983).

Languages act as containers to codify our experience so that it can be captured and conveyed in a form that is somewhat understandable to others and ourselves. However verbal language often structures and limits us as we attempt to place multidimensional experience into conventional linear form. We all have experiences beyond words that are hard to communicate, to ourselves and to others.

Communication in psychotherapy can be seen as a process of transforming inner private subjective experiences and thoughts into external public form. There, in the context of an interpersonal relationship, formerly subjective knowledge becomes accessible to recognition and validity in a shared consensual world. This communication does not always have to be done with verbal language alone. The opportunity exists for expression of attitudes, feelings, ideations and images at a nonverbal level. Such communication can be of considerable value in the psychotherapeutic process and in understanding the 'frame of reference' of the other. Nonverbal experiences, in addition to being of communicative value, can create for the individual an opportunity to find more expedient expressions and gratifications of basic needs. Work at the nonverbal level can lead to new concepts of self and the world. Sandtray World Play can be seen as a tool of expression, which when chosen by the client within the Person-Centered Approach, can facilitate conceptualization of nonverbal, multidimensional aspects of a person's organismic felt sense.

Person Centered Approach

The Person Centered Approach is an approach to counseling, education, organizational development, and a way of being based on the work of psychotherapist Carl Rogers (1902-1987). Rogers' work is concerned with understanding the frame of reference of the other person, as well as understanding the uniqueness of our own, and to appreciate these differences (Brazier, 1993). This approach adopts the belief that the client is the one who possesses the resources for change, having the worth, dignity and the capacity for self-direction. Rather than managing symptoms the Person-Centered Approach emphasizes a stance that creates a climate for growth from within individuals.

In practice, this emphasizes the therapist's role as being empathetic, open and honest, authentic and caring as she listens in depth and facilitates the authenticity of the client. Based on a trust in an inherent impulse toward growth in every individual the therapist relies upon the client for the direction that therapy takes. But not every statement of a client receives equal attention (Rogers, 1970). Person-centered therapists are generally more interested in the meanings and feelings of a client's experience rather than on details of circumstances that lead to their experiences.

A trust in the individual's ability to understand and re-mediate their own problems is at the core of the Person Centered Approach. The basic tenants that provide the foundations for this approach to therapeutic work is stated briefly by Rogers (1980, p.115), "individuals have within themselves vast resources for self-understanding and for altering their self-concepts, basic attitudes, and self-directed behavior; these resources can be tapped if a definable climate of facilitative psychological attitudes can be provided". According to Rogers, the necessary climate that releases our formative, or actualizing tendency is characterized by three attitudes of the therapist: congruence, unconditional positive regard, and empathy (1959, 1980).

Over the years, there has been a growing diversity within the person-centered community. The therapeutic philosophy with its core values has been implemented in a variety of ways. For the most part this change in technique has not necessarily meant a violation of the basic philosophy. Sandtray therapy can certainly be considered person-centered while creating a climate of genuineness, empathy and unconditionality as the bases for understanding and relating to individuals, families or groups. An egalitarian, experiential relationship in that sense also reflects a therapist's readiness to accept corrections by clients (Brink, 1996).

Sandtray World Play

Sandtray is not a new school of therapy but rather a therapeutic tool that provides access to the dynamic and drama of life in miniature (Stone, 1980). The Sandtray apparatus consists of a wooden tray filled with dry or wet sand. The tray is used in combination with an extensive collection of miniature objects that are used to create a scene within the tray. In so doing, sand and objects are used spontaneously to create images and pictures that can then become the vehicle for personal awareness and interpersonal communication.

Play with sand, water, miniature and natural objects in a tray, was frequently used as a therapeutic tool in Europe during the first half of the century. In the 1920's, Margaret Lowenfeld in London developed the use of Sandtray in the psychotherapeutic treatment of children (Lowenfeld, 1939). She found that conventional language is limited in its capacity to stand for uniquely individual experiences. The multidimensional nature of sandtray—that goes beyond time, space and linear logic—seemed to be ideally suited for the type of psychological thinking and meaning making that occurs in the psychic life of children. Lowenfeld realized that children think in experientially vivid images, not words or archetypes. Sandtray play allowed for the emergence of this experiential thinking process. In Switzerland, Dora Kalff (1987), a Jungian analyst, adopted Sandtray for her work with clients in the service of the individuation process as described by Jung. Sandtray therapy was found to accelerate the verbal and nonverbal workings of the Jungian analysis.

Most recently, in the United States, Gisela Schubach De Domenico has developed Sandtray as a psychotherapeutic tool that is verbally independent, requiring neither artistic, mechanical nor specific linguistic skills. She emphasizes that sandtray play facilitates dynamic creative exploration and experimentation (De Domenico, 1988). Sandtray play allows the psyche of each client to determine the course of psychotherapy. The therapist learns how to join the client's psyche. De Domenico stresses that Sandtray is an expressive approach to psychological healing and transformation that is self-guided by the client (1992). The fact that it is also spontaneous, verbally independent, and does not rely on conventional linear, analytical logic allows both client and therapist access to the deepest layers of human awareness. It facilitates personal growth, heals through conscious and creative re-experiencing, and teaches words for experiences that have been labeled as inaccessible, nonexistent or unconscious by family and society.

Using sandtray, the client is able to translate personal experiences into the verbal realm by using sand, water and miniatures. Sandtray World Play is a tool that taps into connections between physical, emotional, mental, social, and spiritual experiences. The client (from hereon also called builder) learns to experience, translate and interpret their own inner and outer world realities as the therapists observes, facilitates, deepens and intensifies these meanings and their connections.

Sandtray Set Up

The sandtray tool consists of one or several waterproof trays made out of wood, plastic or any other waterproof material. The tray is the receptive container in which the client expresses. The trays for individual or couple work are approximately 20 inches by 24 inches and 3 inches deep. Each tray is placed on a waist high work surface. The trays are filled halfway with either moist or dry fine sand: 0-30 mesh white or natural silica sand. Different color and textures of sand may be considered. Water is made available for flooding and water play.

The trays, sand and water are used in conjunction with an extensive collection of miniatures of all kinds, with a diversity of objects, colors and sizes. The miniatures are sorted on shelves according to categories; prehistoric, wild and domestic animals, shells, stones and trees, birds and insects, vehicles for transportation, houses, a full range of male and female figures of different ages, as well as religious and fantasy reproductions. In addition to a general collection, it is important to include objects of particular significance to certain client populations, for instance figures with ethnic diversity, working devices such as computers, and miniatures that resemble groups.

The builder of the Sandtray world uses the sand and objects freely and spontaneously within the tray to create images and pictures that can then become the vehicle for personal awareness and interpersonal communication. Sandtray images correspond to the uniquely individual realities of the builder and are not expected to meet theoretical, clinical, realistic or artistic standards of any kind. Throughout the process of building the therapist (from hereon interchangeably called witness-observer or companion) receives the sandtray creations with an attitude of unconditional positive regard, witnessing and honoring them as deeply meaningful expressions of the psychic life of their creator.

Person-Centered Sandtray

When based upon the foundational belief of the actualizing tendency and an awareness of the necessary conditions of empathy, genuineness and unconditionality, Sandtray provides a framework for the person-centered therapeutic process as described by Rogers in his founding book Counseling and Psychotherapy. Rogers suggested that the therapeutic contact itself is a growth experience. "Here the individual learns to understand himself, to make significant independent choices, to relate to himself successfully to another person." he states (1942, p.30). Looking at this growth experience process in client-centered therapy he consistently witnessed a sequence of steps. He was careful to acknowledge that these steps are not all discrete events but shade into each other and the order he describes is an approximation. After outlining the sequence, Rogers cited an early study supportively consistent with his observations. Taken as a study of the journey of change and progression in the process of person centered therapy these steps can be grouped into five broader stages

(Barrett-Lennard, 1990) which correspond to the stages of Sandtray World Play.

Entering the Process, Building the World

Rogers saw the first stage of therapy as entering into the process. The helping situation is defined, verbally and non-verbally. From the first the client is aware that here is a safe place where his problems can be expressed and he can work out his own solutions. Rogers emphasizes that the beginning stage includes the dawning awareness that what the client thinks and feels matter to the therapist and that is the essential agenda of person-centered therapy. A client's free expression is encouraged by an accepting and receptive attitude. Intellectual explanation is not sufficient (Rogers, 1942).

In Sandtray, the play of the builder is allowed to unfold, moving from critical, rational consciousness to the experience of sensation and the power of the imagination. The power of the imagination and its connection to reality unite while activating the emotions and feelings from the images in the sand picture.

After showing the client the materials that may be worked with the client is invited to either work with the sand for a while and to see what will happen or to do whatever he is tempted to do. Clients may also utilize art materials to build their own figures. It is essential that the builder actually understands that he may freely and spontaneously use all materials in any way he wishes. Whatever the builder wants the materials to be, they are. There is no right or wrong way of using them; there is only the builder's way. Neither the client nor the therapist knows where this experience will lead nor are decisions made in advance as to what contents will be explored.

While the client builds or plays with the materials provided the therapist-observer does not engage in interaction, either physically or verbally but attends with full presence, witnesses with unconditional respect, compassion and awareness. The builder lets the therapist know when the building is completed. Having finished the World, the builder stands or sits in front of the images in the sandtray. He begins to "own" her World by giving it time to let it move her. In so facing her creation, the World might confront the builder but the therapist does not. Sitting with the builder, the therapist receives the client and the World in a nonverbal accepting of the client's journey.

The task for the therapist-companion during the sandtray process is complex. The therapist provides the environment as well as the materials for the sandtray play. The ease and openness with which the needs of the client are accepted and addressed is the first of many nonverbal communications between therapist and client. In addition to providing a safe atmosphere, the therapist needs to be fully attentive to each activity of the builder as he creates his world. Because the first phase of sandtray building is done without discussion the therapist-witness tunes into the pace, the movements, the breath, the face, the being of the client beyond words. The therapist's attending occurs on multiple levels.

The most obvious task involves the factual observer who notices and records the manner in which objects are chosen, rejected, combined and rearranged. This focused observation and attention frequently has a profound healing effect on clients of all ages, eventually helping them to consider their thoughts, actions, feelings and creations as serious and important not only to themselves but to others. The physical pose of attention, observing, note taking, and sketching of the World building process models receptivity, respect and caring. It is an act of body communication from the therapist/witness/companion to the builder. The builder, whose personal creative strivings might have often been ignored or belittled by significant others frequently undergoes a powerful corrective experience when the therapist observes the creative process and refrains from critiquing or correcting the work. Judgment does not always take the form of criticism. Approval is another form of judgment and although it hurts less than criticism clients might be harmed in far more subtle ways. Approval still constitutes an exterior locus of evaluation. For real growth it is as nourishing as cotton candy. Yet, people might spend their lives pursuing it.

That the therapist-observer actually records and documents the process is often an indication to the builder that the work is of enduring value. That the therapist takes time to deeply take notice of the client's smallest move without being intrusive or judgmental facilitates the builder to become aware of herself. Witnessing the sand tray building process is highly essential for the client as well as for the therapist. By simply observing the creation of the world the therapist is much more likely to appreciate the richness of each unique part of the World of the other. This way one truly respects the World and can begin to enter into its mysteries with its builder. No words substitute for the in-depth, primarily nonverbal, observational experience. The witness-companion begins to provide the psychologically safe container for the sandtray, the builder and the emerging World. The witness-companion models that the activity of the moment has intrinsic meaning.

Deepening in Dialogue

In the second stage of therapy accepting, recognizing and clarifying the experiences of the client whatever their nature, is of central importance to Rogers. "The counselor's whole function at this stage is to encourage free expression" and "to create an atmosphere in which the client can come to recognize that he has these feelings and can accept them" (Rogers, 1942, p.36, 38). The centrality of feeling and expression is sustained and deepened with the communication of the experience to another. Movement in the client's experience, which the therapist has been continually reflecting and clarifying, becomes more visible during this time. During this stage, experience may have a chaotic quality because the patient has entered his own world of unresolved experiences and touched untapped raw energy.

As the process moves on, Rogers notes that there is a resolution of present problems to varying degrees. This, in turn, seems to release more energy, which enables a still deeper look into the individual's experience. The dark, unwanted energies, when given room, lead the way toward more constructive, positive impulses which make for growth. Rogers emphasizes that these positive feelings are accepted as no more and no less a part of the personality than the negative ones. It is this total acceptance of the all aspects of the person's World that gives the individual an opportunity for the first time in his life to understand himself as he is. "He has no need to be defensive about his negative feelings. He is given no opportunity to overvalue his positive feelings. And in this type of situation, insight and self understanding come bubbling through spontaneously" (Rogers, 1942, p.40).

The second stage is transformative for the client according to De Domenico (1994). When given acceptance and room, previously frightening images in a person's experience begin to evolve into resources that he uses to transform old, mechanical behaviors into new, life-enhancing responses.

During this joint experiencing phase the therapist joins the client in front of the sandtray and asks to be taken into the world. The World is fully experienced from the perspective of the builder. The builder now verbalizes the experiences contained in the World, so that they may both talk about the World and how it is. The client is the expert and the guide. The therapist-observer travels through the World with the builder. The sandtray is viewed form all sides. Prepositional and relational placements are noticed. Without getting lost in details, the part and the whole are both contained. Verbal reflections by the therapist further deepen and intensify the builder's capacity to observe and experience the World confronting him.

The Sandtray therapist who asks to be introduced to the world of the builder needs to trust the client's actualization. She has to answer the following hypothetical questions faithfully before she can enter a builder's world as a trustworthy companion: Is the inner experience of the client benign or dangerous? Is the therapist able to respect that the builder is the expert of the World about to be entered?, Is the therapist aware of her personal, subjective experiences evoked by the World of the client? Can the therapist be the innocent who, following the wisdom of the client's knowing, asks apparently simple questions about the beings and happenings in the World?

When the therapist-companion trusts the wisdom of the builder's psyche they can both explore the Sandtray that provides a three dimensional view of the client's world. The boundaries of the tray are physical reminders of personal and psychological boundaries. Only the builder touches or moves figures in the tray and it is the builder who knows the meaning and character of objects in the World. Only the builder knows what is true within the wooden frame. The therapist enters the evolving World as an empathetic companion to the actively experiencing builder. This witness-companion allows herself to wonder in awe, assuming nothing. She allows herself to be curious about the building process, about the meaning and purpose of each figurine, and what it would be like to live in this World. The therapist's phenomenological experience, when fully present in the evolving sandtray world, can validate the builder's experience. The therapist-companion simultaneously adds her eyes, ears, kinesthetic sense, her physical body and emotional body, her symbolic as well as logical experiencing to that of the client. Entering into the client's world with love, compassion and awareness the therapist strives to see and connect with the wholeness of the Other before her. Being seen in such a manner opens the client to seeing more of himself and his experience. Exploring and communicating one's world in dialogue with a benevolent witness-companion thereby deepens a person's unique experience of himself or herself.

Insight and Wholeness

Eventually, Rogers postulated that the client reaches a stage of insight, understanding of the self and acceptance of the self. Intermingled with this process of insight is a process of clarification of possible decisions and possible courses of action. The client has a sense of having "touched home", of reaching wholeness. A paradoxical change occurs. By surrendering to his inner wisdom and embodying it the person gains a new sense of order and security and a new sense of his own worth.

Sandtray, as a tool of expression, allows the client to view his world in an over seeable, tangible form. His reality, in metaphor, with all of its complexities, conflicts and paradoxes is held within one frame. It is possible to literally move his body to view aspects of her World from new previously hidden angles and perspectives. The Worlds itself confronts the maker not the therapist. This multisensorial overview facilitates new awareness and insight on the part of the builder. Although the builder cannot simultaneously verbalize all aspects of her process, he has the possibility to hold the entire experience in awareness by simply regarding the objects. The gap in experience of the body, emotion and mind is more easily bridged as it is all held in the sandtray as one complete system. It provides a means of conveying images and their meaning directly and simultaneously that might not be so easily communicated. Individuals, families or groups can gain a new sense of integrating aspects of preverbal experience and verbal modes of communication during the sandtray process and the exploratory discussion that follows.

After experiencing and processing their World with a therapist-companion, builders reflect on what they believe the message of the World is. They ponder the wisdom that their experience is providing through the free and spontaneous expression in the sand thereby integrating newly gained insights.

Taking the Meaning into Daily Life

Rogers stated that the client who has gained an understanding of himself to a degree which enables him to take positive steps in the light of her new orientation needs to take that learning into the world.

In the fourth stage of Sandtray, therapy the wholeness experienced and expressed through sand must now find its expressions in the wholeness of living. The new insight emerging from the sandtray experience has to be experimented with in the outside world by the builder. Rogers observed that the insight and tentative positive movements in therapy lead to more complete and accurate self-understanding which leads to increasingly integrated positive action on the part of the client. The client decides if and how he wishes the sandplay to be photographed. These photos may be used in later sessions. Photos preserve some aspect of the healing journey and are frequently a meaningful reminder of the session for the client. Occasionally the client will give the photograph a title, further emphasizing what has been learned during the play. The photos and words can be taken as a reminder into the client's life outside of the therapy room. Translating the complex, multisensorial, multidimensional experience into some form of linear expression is an important part of remembering and carrying the learnings of the sandtray session into life outside of the therapy session. By attempting to summarize or capture the message of the World the client is better able to assimilate, in cognitive form, an experience that might otherwise remain too abstract to utilize in the outside world. The seemingly simple act of photographing and naming the World becomes an important part of translating the sandtray experience into a valid part of the client's memory and long-term world view.

Termination and Dismantling the Builder's World

Rogers saw the final stage of therapy as the recognition and gradual acceptance on the part of the client that the therapy relationship must end. He pointed out that there is also a feeling of decreasing need for continuing help.

Sandtray offers several ways of terminating therapy or dismantling the builder's world. Sometimes a tray is left to stand undisturbed until the next meeting with the client when work on the Sandtray world is continued. At other times it is important for the builder to leave the World intact and whole after the session is finished, even if the client will not return to work on that particular tray in the future. In such a case the client is offered the possibility that the therapist will dismantle the sandplay after the builder has left the room. No one handles the builder's world in front of her since that could violate the client's experience.

In most cases, the builder dismantles her own tray when the session is finished. When the builder does the dismantling, it is a meaningful expression and experience of endings. The builder is the one who "breaks the energy pattern" of the intact World. The builder then removes and returns figures to their original place on the shelves and smooths out the sand. The meaningfulness has now shifted from the World build in sand to the personhood of the client.

Conclusion

Sometimes, more than one Sandtray session might be needed to support a person's transformational process. Nevertheless, each session is a whole and complete transformational process in and by itself. Rogers suggested this about person-centered therapy when he proposed that therapy is not a preparation for change, rather it *is* change (1942, p.30). During therapy a new pattern of change and adjustment is experienced and laid down. Transformation and healing occurs in the process of acquiring new insights and taking them into daily life.

The Sandtray process creates a bridge between the internalized imagery of the world of experience and the externalized manifestation of this experience, a bridge between the nonverbal and verbal, between tacit and direct knowing. Sandtray World Play allows both client and therapist to reach deep multidimensional levels of experiencing while providing images to facilitate the verbally independent language of being. It is a dynamic approach to creative exploration of the client's world. Sandtray based on person-centered principles provides a means of effective counseling which

Rogers described as "a definitely structured, permissive relationship which allows the client to gain an understanding of himself to a degree which enables him to take positive steps into the light of his new orientation" (1942, p.18). Sandtray used as an integral part of the therapeutic process seems to facilitate—even accelerate—this journey into Self. The experiential tool provides a container for positive human experiences that are also intellectually meaningful. The playful ambiance of an overseeable, self-created world allows for a genuine focus on a person's experience and his unique potential to re-mediate his problems.

Susan & Joachim Schwarz are affiliated with the Center for the Studies of the Person in LaJolla, CA.

References

Barrett-Lennard, G. (1990). The therapy pathway reformulated. In Lietaer, Rombauts, Van Balen (Eds.) **Client-centered and experiential psychotherapy in the nineties**. Leuven, Belgium: Leuven University Press.

Brazier, D. (1993). **Beyond Carl Rogers**. London: Constable and Company Limited.

Brink, D. (1996). Rogers' therapy cases. In B. Farber, D. Brink, P. Raskin (Eds.) **The psychology of Carl Rogers: Cases and commentary**. New York: The Guilford Press.

De Domenico, G. (1988). **Sandtray world play: a comprehensive guide to the use of the sand tray in psychotherapeutic and transformational settings**. Oakland: Vision Quest.

De Domenico, G. (1992). **Sand Tray World Play training: and introduction to the art of sandtray therapy**. Oakland: Vision Quest.

Frank, J. (1973). **Persuasion and healing: A comparative study of psychotherapy** (rev. ed.). Baltimore: John Hopkins University Press.

Frank, J. (1987). Psychotherapy, rhetoric, and hermeneutics: Implications for practice and research. **Psychotherapy, 24**, 293-302.

Horvath, P. (1988). Placebos and common factors in two decades of psychotherapy research. **Psychological Bulletin, 104**, 214-225.

Kalff, D. (1987). **Sandplay: a psychotherapeutic approach to the psyche**. Boston: Sigo Press.

Lowenfeld, M. (1939). The world pictures of children: a method of recording and studying them. **The British Journal of Medical Psychology, 18**(1),

Prioleau, L., Murdock, M., & Brody, N. (1983). An analysis of psychotherapy versus placebo studies. **The Behavioral and Brain Sciences, 6**, 275-310.

Rogers, C.R. (1942). **Counseling and psychotherapy**. Boston: Houghton Mifflin.

Rogers, C.R. (1959). A theory of therapy, personality, and interpersonal relationships, as developed in the client-centered framework. In S. Koch (Ed.), **Psychology: a study of science**. New York: McGraw Hill.

Rogers, C.R. (1980). **On encounter groups**. New York: Harper & Row.

Rogers, C.R. (1980). **A way of being**. Boston: Houghton Mifflin.

Stone, H. (1980). Prologue. In Kalff (Ed.) **Sandplay: a psychotherapeutic approach to the psyche**. Boston: Sigo Press.

Zilbergeld, B. (1983). **The shrinking of America: Myths of psychological change**. New York: Little, Brown.

Applications of the Person-centered Approach in Health Care: Helping Health Care Care

David Meador

Despite escalating expenditures and remarkable advances, Americans seem to be expressing their distrust of the health care system at higher and higher levels. I believe that patients are missing, longing for, the feeling of being given the sort of care that comes with rich human contact. They want to feel as though they as individuals are more important than the system. Modern medicine has unknowingly created quite a dilemma for itself. In its highly admirable race to find cures for all sorts of diseases, it has let its patients down in a very personal and important way. Patients want to believe that they are highly valued as individuals. If that is not their perception, then let's change that. We have a lot of good people providing health care and we have the psycho-social tools to help them be more effective healers. What are we waiting for?

Many physicians, nurses and other health care professionals seem to know, perhaps intuitively, how to build genuinely warm and nourishing relationships with those under their care. This extraordinary type of relationship is a fundamental element in the successful treatment of the whole person. Though knowledgeable as they are in their area of expertise, most will benefit from something akin to personal awareness "training" or personal growth groups to be able to establish the sort of relationships that are fulfilling and effective for themselves, their patients and coworkers. I believe that the person-centered approach to such group work is most appropriate.

I was first invited in 1991 to help staff the week long Winter Course of The American Academy on Physician and Patient. AAPP is made up largely of medical school faculty and is dedicated to the idea that medical education should include in its curriculum courses that will promote and enhance the interpersonal relationship skills that the physician brings to the relationship with the patient. It was then that I started to focus on the quality of the relationship between the health care system and its professionals as well as with the patient and the process of healing.

Relationship and Healing

Medical technology seems to have developed a will of its own and is challenging the role of the physician as healer. Most medical students enter formal education with their ideals in place and a bright vision of themselves as healers. Then the process we call medical education slowly erodes that precious mission. Sadly, success in medical school has little to do with the ability to develop a healing relationship and much to do with learning exceedingly sophisticated technologies. Both doctor and patient are cheated.

America is graying. As we feel our physical vulnerabilities, our concerns about raising health care costs abound. There is a general unease felt about our current health care system. I believe an intentional effort to restore that original and valid impulse to heal is highly appropriate at this time.

No one comes out of medical school without scars. The physical and emotional stress that such training demands will have its effect. A necessary ingredient to strengthening or restoring a physician's healing instincts is to provide occasions for emotional healing and growth. It is cruelly ironic that there are so few institutionalized opportunities for the healing of the healers.

In order for physicians to feel fulfilled in their practice, they must feel effective. A corner stone in the practice of the healing arts is the doctor/patient relationship. Unless a physician is able to offer the patient genuine warmth and openness, the relationship will remain limited to the realm of techno-treatment. Stress and self doubt greatly diminish one's ability to offer these heartfelt qualities to others.

In his Book, Peace, Love & Healing (1990), Bernie S. Siegel, M.D., writes:

The doctor I would want for myself or anyone else I cared about would be one who understands that disease is more than just a clinical entity; it is an experience and a metaphor, with a message that must be listened to...Only by listening to that message can we mobilize all the healing powers that lie within, and that is what the doctor must help each patient do. (p. 119)

Emmett E. Miller, M.D., writing in Healers on Healing (1989) asserts:

Two crucial requirements of the healing process are trust and honesty. By trust I mean that both the healer and the person to be healed have confidence that there is a power within the body that has the capacity to bring about healing when it is given the opportunity to do so. By honesty I mean the healer's willingness to be faithful and true to the spirit of the patient. In my practice I have seen how both of these qualities must be present for any genuine healing to occur. They are key strands in the golden thread that binds together all methods of healing. (p. 119)

Each time the patient is offered a relationship that is perceived as caring, honest and genuinely accepting, a movement toward greater self knowledge and an enhanced feeling of self worth will emerge. This quality of relationship is the basis of effective psychotherapy.

While I am not suggesting that health care providers take on the additional role of psychotherapist, I do believe that enhancing their relationship skills will be beneficial to the healing process. Deepening the quality of the relationship will allow the care giver greater insight into how the disease process is related to the patient's life experience. I would expect that this enriched level of understanding and knowledge about the patient to be personally rewarding for the care giver.

Nourishing Healers

Many physicians have reported to me that they have benefited from participating in a small groups I have facilitated using the Person-Centered Approach. Insights into their style of relating to patients, and others, has allowed them to become more effective and satisfied in their practice. Since 1978 the American Academy on Physician and Patient, has used PCA small group work as one of its central educational tools. Mack Lipkin, Jr., M.D., past president of AAPP explains in brochure entitled Listening, learning, teaching:

The medical interview relies for its success on a genuine and empathic response on the part of the physician. The personal awareness groups challenge each individual to explore the emotional strengths and resources he or she brings to the medical encounter.

Penny Williamson, Sc.D., a former Academy vice president writes about physician support groups:

A comprehensive definition of professionalism ought to reflect our universal need for sharing and connectedness with others; and the recognition that such sharing provides an avenue for understanding oneself, as well as one's peers, patients, students and significant others. Physicians are responsible for more than technical knowledge. They must also develop in-depth self knowledge. It is the combination of technical and self knowledge which transforms the physician from technician to healer (my emphasis)...Self knowledge is harder to achieve in isolation than in group settings where individuals are helped to see themselves as others see them. Support groups provide a safe forum for participants to reveal feelings and explore various aspects of being a physician. (p. 180)

I use the person-centered approach to facilitate personal awareness groups and find that it is very powerful and effective in a wide variety of settings and with very diverse populations. One key of this approach to group leadership is for the facilitator to help create an atmosphere of safety and acceptance within the group. The facilitator moves the group forward by striving to be an authentic participant and caring group member with well developed listening skills. By allowing the group process to evolve at its own rate, it is assured that participants can come to be known to each other at a pace that is appropriate for and respectful of who they are.

As members of a personal awareness group get to know one another and they begin to trust that it is safe to be known on a deep level, strong bonds of support develop. Many participants report feeling more secure about being the person they genuinely are than they ever have before. A closeness and sense of community develops. They come to learn that openness, honesty and feelingful expression can be beneficial when appropriate.

Participants find themselves becoming empowered and their new found community also develops a very positive potency. Out of a sense of self acceptance and self worth a physician will emerge better able to easily establish the type of healing relationships with their patients of which they had once dreamed.

The Healing Environment

I think it is unfair, given the horrendous demands of medical training and of the field in general, to expect the medical profession to be able to be all things to all patients. However, it seems to me that by modifying the psycho-social environment of our hospitals and clinics it would be possible to cultivate a type of supportive psychological environment that would encourage nourishing relationships for the givers and recipients of health care.

In many hospitals there seems to be a degree of stress that goes with the job. In addition to feeling "over worked and under paid," there is often a feeling of being under appreciated. This can be as true for a chief nurse as for an orderly. A hierarchy of status and power contributes to tensions among staff and with the physicians.

Some hospitals are not safe places to seek psychological support or express personal needs. They can and should be.

In order for practitioners and other care givers to be able to offer nourishing relationships to their patients and each other, they themselves need to be nourished. By creating an atmosphere of shared trust and personal awareness, a staff will emerge that will be better able to work together for the benefit of their patients and institution.

Nourishing the Organization

The building of a highly supportive psychological community among the staff must be given a high priority. It will be the bed rock from which will spring the sort of nourishing attitudes that are crucial to the type of healing environment I am envisioning. There are applications within the Person-Centered Approach that can promote psychological community in an organization. It is not a particularly fast paced process when applied within a work setting, but it can work. It may bring about dynamic change and it will be resisted by some. Others will welcome it.

I particularly value the Person-Centered Approach (PCA) because it is always respectful of the individual(s) and the organization with whom it is being applied. PCA helps individuals and organizations move in a self selected direction. When individuals and the group aggregate feel satisfied that their personal ideas and needs are fully understood, they are likely to be somewhat open to a journey into community.

When making an intervention into the dynamics of an organization it is important to have institutional support at as many levels as possible. The advantages to the organization must be understood. A mutually agreed upon mission must be articulated. Positive personal outcomes must be envisioned by its leaders. When organizational support is not widespread, it may be possible to do a demonstration project within a department.

When beginning organizational development work, I believe a "needs and wants" survey that looks for areas of satisfaction and of dissatisfaction is a good way to initiate the process. Participants are then invited to meet in small, facilitated groups to discuss the survey results. While no ongoing work group is without some form of hierarchy, sometimes in the early stages of this work I have found it best to meet with groups made up of people of similar rank. A dynamic grid of issues will emerge encompassing areas of concern from within and out of the group.

Over the course of several meetings a climate of increased trust will emerge allowing for more personal issues to be expressed. This will foster a supportive atmosphere that will allow for a feeling of relative closeness. Honest feedback will be exchanged within the relative safety of the group. Often the participants will recognize the advantage to themselves and to their work that this experience affords and choose to continue meeting on a regular basis.

As more groups are formed within the organization, a networking among groups may emerge addressing areas of common concern. Surprisingly creative solutions often are found for problems that had once seemed unapproachable. Eventually, a sufficient number of groups and individuals will discover shared needs and goals. A heightened degree of trust will allow for mutually beneficial problem solving. A personal accountability for self satisfaction and job performance will contribute to creativity and organizational efficiency.

Nourishing the Patient and Family

This same group process can be very helpful for the patient. Hospitalization can be very lonely, stressful and disorienting; hardly qualities that promote healing. In the Archives of General Psychiatry, Fawzy, F., Cousins, N., et al. report:

Despite the prevailing belief that patients with early stages of cancer and with a good prognoses should have "nothing to worry about," it is apparent that patients with newly diagnosed cancer, regardless of their prognosis, exhibit symptoms of psychological distress similar to those of patients undergoing bone marrow transplantation as a last resort treatment of leukemia, patients with AIDS and other patients with cancer in general. (p. 722)

An appropriate level of group participation may have a tremendous impact on the healing process from the time of diagnosis and continuing as long as the patient finds it beneficial. It has been demonstrated that participation in support groups seems to have dramatically increased the life expectancy of some cancer patients. (Spiegel D. & Bloom J., 1989) But, survival rates aside, a warm and supportive psychological community can have a tremendous positive impact on the quality of life for the patient, family and loved ones. Anxiety and depression are common symptoms of hospitalization. Being able to discuss these issues in a supportive environment typically reduces their negative impact upon both patient and staff.

Another opportunity to impact well-being lies with the patient's significant others. Illness is stressful for this group, too. Often it is difficult for a patient's family and friends to express freely the fears, concern, anger, love and confusion that are prompted by a serious illness. The patient and the loved ones often believe it is important to protect each other from intense or new feelings. This is most unfortunate and leads to a stressful alienation for the patient. The use of PCA support groups with this population may have tremendous immediate and long term effects on the wellness of the patient and loved ones.

Treating the Untreatable

Experts estimate that as many as 60 percent or more of people's visits to doctors are for health problems that elude diagnosis or do not respond to traditional medical treatment. This remarkable observation is found on the web site of harvardpilgrim healthcare, one of this nations most highly respected HMO.

There is increasing concern, especially in HMOs, about the drain of resources that results from the somatizing patient. These patients suffer from a persistent physical discomfort that defies diagnosis and treatment. It is believed that this process occurs when a patient is unable to express psychological distress in any way other than as a physical symptom.

Because these patients experience their pain in an entirely physical context, they resist referral to mental health providers. Further more, the suggestion by the physician that there may be an emotional component to the disease is often taken by the patient as a personal rejection. Frustration, anger, and a sense of helplessness are often experienced by both the physician and patient.

Frederick G. Guggenheim, M.D., Professor of Psychiatry at the University of Arkansas, writes in Somatoform Disorders (1997), "Treatment involves close follow-up by the primary care physician with support of the patient by making inquiry into psychosocial stressors during the episodic exacerbations that these patients suffer associated with their increased emotional tensions" (p. 10). Group work with somatizing patients that augments the medical intervention has been shown to be of significant help in reducing demands on the primary provider. Of perhaps greater importance, the group process would provide opportunities for the patient to safely become aware of emotional issues previously unidentified. This gain in self awareness would mediate physical systems and improve healthfulness generally.

A strategy for willing and successful participation in such a group should include a strong medical component. It can be described as a "disease management" group and its participants need not be limited to those with somatic symptoms. A physician or other medical practitioner should be present during the first session in order to emphasize that this is offered conjointly. In the same vein it would be beneficial if the group work was done in the same setting or building that the physician is practicing in. Sending a patient to another facility sends the message that the patient doesn't really have a medical problem.

Topics such as pain management, disability coping skills and nutrition should be covered, among others. Any topic in a group with a Person-Centered Approach facilitator will provide ample opportunities to explore personal and emotional issues. I have no doubt that this type of cost effective intervention can have a tremendous positive impact on the well being of somatizing patients.

Harvard Pilgrim has designed and implemented an innovative approach to treating this population. The Personal Health Improvement Program (PHIP) is designed for people who have difficulty functioning or exhibit unproductive interpersonal behaviors; have stress related symptom; who are learning to deal with a chronic disease; or whose stress adversely impacts their health.

According to Steven Locke, M.D., chief of behavioral medicine at Harvard Pilgrim, PHIP participants learn to become aware of how they usually respond to stress in daily life and how this affects their health, and are taught new and positive behaviors to deal with these situations. The six-week, six-session program, which is taught by a trained facilitator in small groups, uses interactive exercises, readings, home study, and class discussions to teach skills such as self and body awareness, relaxation, meditation, effective communication, stress management, and mood management.

"Decades of research on how mind and body interactions relate to health—for example, stress and its effects on the heart—are now firmly supported by the findings of psychoneuroimmunology (a field of medicine bringing together psychology, neurology, and immunology)," says Steven Locke, MD, a psychiatrist and director of PHIP at Harvard Pilgrim Health Care. (Moini, S. 1998, web site)

The Healing Facility of the Future

This may be an opportune time to suggest some health care alternatives to complement modern technological interventions. A study done by Harvard internist David Eisenberg, et al., (1993) found that a third of

Americans surveyed had used at least one "unconventional therapy" in the past year. Unconventional therapies were defined as "commonly used interventions neither taught widely in U.S. medical schools nor generally available in U.S. hospitals" (p. 1200).

Modern American hospitals and medical clinics are wonderful places to find exceedingly sophisticated diagnostic and treatment technologies. They are staffed by highly trained and dedicated personnel. The physical environments are clean and usually cheerily decorated. Unfortunately these facilities are often perceived as impersonal by patients and stressful by staff.

The Planetree Model Hospital Project at San Francisco's Pacific Medical Center is an example of how a special healing unit can be incorporated into a traditional hospital. Today planetree has twenty hospitals affiliates in the us and two in Europe. Patients in a Planetree unit enjoy a much more home-like atmosphere where they can sleep as late as they wish and even prepare their own meals if they like. Patients may study their own charts, research their illness in the medical library and participate fully in treatment decisions. "According to Dr. John Gamble, chief of medicine at Pacific Presbyterian Medical Center…'All our research and experience indicate that the incorporation of modern medicine and technology in a setting that upholds the full rights and dignity of the individual patient will add immeasurably to the healing'" (Greer, 1986, p. 70).

An awareness is emerging that a disease involves more than a strictly physical process, but rather also has something to do with a patient's beliefs, life style and self concept. The healing facility of the future will place greater emphasis on treating the whole person. It will be a place where some people may go expecting to be healed in ways that are less limited to a particular medical problem and more generally specific to how they are experiencing life.

The quality of the social environment in the facility and the personal relationships between patient and care providers will be recognized as important elements in the healing process. The staff in the healing facility of the future will be trained in interpersonal communication skills and given opportunities for personal growth. They will be encouraged to get to know patients and their families as people, on a comfortable, personal basis, as well as professionally.

Patients and their families will be active members on teams with physicians, adjunct therapist and support staff designing together a healing program from a menu of therapies. The adjunct therapies available within the facility may include, but not be limited to, meditation, chiropractic, guided imagery, acupuncture, massage, group and individual psychotherapy, nutritional therapy, biofeedback, movement and art therapy. The quality of the patient-therapist relationship will be of primary importance.

The healing facility of the future will have a peaceful, retreat like atmosphere. It will be relaxed with comfortable accommodations for the patient and adjacent housing for family or friends. It may have inviting grounds containing recreational opportunities such as a spa, pool and walking paths. It will have areas indoors and out that facilitate patients, families, friends and staff getting to know one another. It will have a friendly atmosphere oriented around healthfulness and personal awareness as well as healing.

Some Steps

It seems imperative to me that a system for providing emotional support and personal growth must be an integral part of medical education. Not, as it often is now, an elective opportunity for which the student has not the time.

More and more demands are being made of those staffing medical facilities. Creating an environment that is psychologically safe for staff to be at their emotional best must be given a high priority.

Providing emotional support for patients and families will enhance healing and improve their quality of life. It will increase job satisfaction for the staff as well.

Providing support groups for somatizing patients will reduce demands on the health care system and its care givers. Group participants will have an opportunity to get to know themselves and increase their sense of well-being.

The healing facility of the future will provide a social environment that will cater to the whole person, not only the disease. The concept of healing will broaden.

I have touched on some steps that I believe can help our health care providers deliver the type of care that patients are demanding. The Person-Centered Approach has much to offer to improve the quality of life and service of health care providers. It has been my experience that health care systems are reluctant to undertake the sort of interventions I have suggested. That will continue to be the case until they recognize that it is in everyone's best interest to add 'people care' to health care.

David Meador is a member of the Center for Studies of the Person, co-director of the La Jolla Program and a former director of CSP. He was a student and colleague of Carl Rogers from 1968 until his death in 1987. He is a PCA applications specialist and trainer in a variety of settings.

References

Eisenberg, D., Kessler, R. C., Foster, C., Norlock, F. E., Calkins, D. R., & Delbanco, T. L. (1993), January. In R. Friedman, To the Editor: Unconventional medicine. **New England Journal of Medicine.** 329(16), 1200.

Fawzy, F., Cousins, N., et al. (1990). A structured psychiatric intervention for cancer patients. **The archives of general psychiatry,** 47, 722.

Greer, N. R. (1986). Redesigning health care. **Architecture.** 75(4), 68-70.

Guggenheim, F. G. (1997). Somatoform Disorders. Internet: Available, www.uams.edu/department_of_psychiatry/syllabus/somatoform/somatoform.htm. University of Arkansas for Medical Sciences.

Lipkin, M. (1993). Brochure: Listening, learning, teaching. Task Force on Doctor and Patient, Society of General Internal Medicine.

Miller, E. E. (1989). **Healers on Healing.** New York: St. Martin's Press.

Moini, S. (1998). Healthy mind, healthy body: Understanding the mind/body connection. Internet: Active, www.harvardpilgrim.org/health_library/health_categories/stress/healthy_mind_healthy_body.htm. Harvard Pilgrim Health Care.

Siegel, B. S. (1989). **Peace, love & healing.** New York: Harper & Row.

Spiegel, D. & Bloom, J. R. (1989). Effect of psychosocial treatment on survival of patients with metastatic breast cancer. **Lancet,** 2, 888-891.

Williamson, P. R. (1991). Editorial: Support groups: An important aspect of physician education. **Journal of General Internal Medicine.** 6(2), 179-180.

Working with Clients with a Mental Disability and Their Families in a Person-Centered Way: Challenge for the Belief in the Actualizing Tendency

Elisabeth Zinschitz

In this chapter I examine the importance of the core conditions for working with mentally disabled clients and discuss where we may be challenged in our approach. Furthermore, as a reinforcement for empathic understanding, I consider it helpful to have knowledge of the impact a disability can have on the development of the self, the self-concept and the social competence of the individual. Apart from working with adults in order to help them develop a better life quality, more self-determination, a better self-regulation of their emotions or simply a better self-esteem, we can also work with parents of disabled children in order to facilitate their acceptance and understanding of their child and cope with the disability. This process increases the probability of attaining the positive outcome mentioned above for child with a mental disability in becoming an adult.

The Validity of the Moment
by
Jerold Bozarth
I know not what you will do or become
at this moment or beyond;

286

I know not what I will do except stay with you
at this moment
And be mother, father, sister, brother, friend, child, and lover
at this moment;
I exist for you and with you
at this moment;
I give you all of me
at this moment;
I am you
at this moment;
Take me and use me
at this moment
to be whatever you can become
at this moment and beyond

Those are committed to a person-centered approach do not focus on diagnoses and categories of disorders. This fact is often considered responsible for the paucity of the person-centered literature concerned with specific categories of disorders or problems. Rogers (1951) suggests that when the therapist focuses on diagnosing, the client perceives the therapist as the expert, resulting in dependency on the therapist to be responsible for the change in the client. This dependency leads to an opposite effect of therapy: personal growth.

He admits that for the treatment of an organic illness, the physical diagnosis is absolutely necessary. In the case of a disability the diagnosis is not always a physical one: a paralysis is clearly a physical diagnosis, but what about a cognitive disability?

Apart from the professional field, the expression 'handicap', 'disability' etc. have become labels which are apt to stigmatize people. When I speak about 'mentally disabled' clients I am referring to a category of clients, and this may also be considered as labeling. I have however found that I cannot ignore that my clients have been influenced by their disability in their personal development in some way or other. To ignore that would mean not to consider the individual as a whole.

Thorne (1992) has noted that Rogers identified four qualifications of the therapist when he was working with children, one of which was "psychological knowledge." By this Rogers meant a "thorough basis of human behavior and of its physical and social and psychological determinants" (Thorne, 1992, p. 10). Even though "at least by 1946, he did not consider diagnostic knowledge…necessary for good therapy" (Bozarth, 1998, p. 127), I have found it helpful to reflect upon how a disability may have influenced a person's way of experiencing throughout life. I use the knowledge I have about mental disability, just as I use my knowledge about specific aspects of being a woman, or being a mother or to be living in a country that is not my own, etc. This knowledge does not necessarily reinforce my prejudices or my expectations about a particular individual. It rather reinforces my capacity for empathic understanding, i.e. for trying to understand the internal frames of reference of individuals. Thus, with due respect to the objections to labeling, one cannot escape it.

The way of describing a person who is impaired on an intellectual, physical or sensory level has changed over the years. The word 'handicap' has disappeared because of its negative connotation, the term 'disability' came up and recently the label has evolved to 'person with special needs'. I tend to not use 'person with special needs', because in a way every person has special or specific needs, and even though the boundaries between non-disabled and disabled persons are not always clear, I still am speaking about a specific group with a specific characteristic consisting of an impairment in a certain primary physical or mental ability. I would like to point out that I am not referring here to what is known as 'emotional' or 'social disabilities;' those I consider as 'secondary disabilities' resulting from traumatic childhood experiences—like maltreatment, neglect, abuse—or from an inadequate way of dealing with the primary disability by parents or other caretakers.

Every disability, whether cognitive, physical or other, has an influence on personal development. In this paper, I restrict myself to describing my work with adults who have problems on a cognitive level. I may, however, refer to physical or sensory impairments as examples of the impact these impairments may have on the development of the self-concept.

This paper focuses on psychotherapy with clients who have mental disabilities. However, my experience, as well as other information, have confirmed that the person centered approach is not only effective clientele.

Diagnosis Versus Telling a Personal Story

My use of knowledge about possible implications of a mental disability for personal development remains, however, very tentative. After all, categories offer merely a rough description because they do not include everything; they certainly fail to offer information on the course development will take.

When parents learn that their child is disabled, they most likely are eager to hear from the medical staff how the child will develop. It confuses them when doctors speak in generalities and do not provide a clear perspective. Whoever is not familiar with the issue may tend to think that disability categories are clearly distinguishable and they do not understand until the child grows older that it is hard to draw a straight line. Of course the child's development is impaired on different levels and also stops at certain points. But in other areas each child may develop asynchronously: speech may develop late, and yet the child may seem to have some understanding of what the parents say. The child may be slow in learning, yet on an emotional and social level may be astonishingly skillful. Parents are often surprised repeatedly by their child's learning, which they had already given up on.

When I started to work with young children with disabilities, I also had this concept of disability categories. In a way it was helpful as an instrument which I could use to speak with colleagues about my work, but I soon learned substantially more about development, and how it can take an entirely different course for each individual child, even though each may have the same diagnosis. In psychotherapy, for example, it may be helpful to know that the client who is coming to see me is blind. I can prepare myself to 'show' him the way around in my practice; I am also open to the fact that his experiencing most likely has been influenced by his hearing, and not by his sight. What happens is that I create an image within myself of how the child is groping his way through this world. But upon arrival find an extremely insecure and shaky man. He gives me the impression that the onset of his disability occurred yesterday and he still has to get used to it. His blindness, in combination with the experiences he made being blind, have influenced his development on many levels: his way of thinking, his way of feeling, his speech, his walking and moving. This information teaches me what use I can make of my concept of blindness and where it is not helpful at all. I must be open to whatever comes, and this openness requires some security within myself with respect to people who in many ways are much more different from me than others.

It lies in the nature of human beings that what is unknown, strange, alien to us evokes in us cautiousness, fear and even disgust, and on the other hand also curiosity, interest and fascination. I believe part of our tendency to categorize everything arises out of fear; as a result, we categorize in order to get this fear under control within ourselves in psychotherapy, but can also be useful for caretakers and other professions who work with this. Below a shortened version of how Feuser describes it:

1. Whenever there is something about another person that we cannot understand and which we cannot accept as also relevant or applicable to ourselves, we think that this person is not understandable to us because of his or her different way of being.

2. We can only understand others through projection of the boundaries of our understanding onto this other person, i.e. we think that the boundaries of our understanding are the boundaries of those we have to

understand. That is why we perceive our own boundaries as the boundaries of the other person.

3. Our assumptions about these boundaries of the other person which now we consider as part of his or her way of being make us transfer this person to learning systems as well as to living, working and therapy conditions which correspond to our assumption of his or her boundaries. This guarantees that the person remains the way I am able to imagine him or her. This leads to the fulfillment of our prognosis about his or her possibilities of growth and it affirms us, proves our 'normality' and his or her 'pathology'. This way the circle remains unbroken. (Feuser, p. 6)

In professional literature on disability one always finds categories of disabilities, like sensory impairment, physical disability, mental deficiency etc. It is true, in practice, that sometimes a disability is clearly and correctly described by such a label. In general however the dividing-line between these categories is blurred. And that is understandable because one step in human development implies the next and so they are connected. For example, a lack of hearing leads to impaired vocal speech and may also be associated with difficulties in developing a notion of abstract ideas. If a baby does not learn how to grasp objects, as it usually does from the age of four months, it may have problems in grasping other things on a cognitive level. The fact that a child is paralyzed can influence other aspects in the development of his personality. As Müller-Breckwoldt and Lipinski who worked in a person-centered way with a group of children with spina bifida, have noted:

It is possible that the fact that they cannot take one step on their own without being inhibited may limit the consciousness of life, may make the individuation of the child and his or her growth towards a unique individual that wants to develop his or her capacities considerably more difficult. It is very likely that the self-concept of these children is strongly influenced by their deficits and that this is reinforced by an environment which very often draws its first impression from the 'abnormal' appearance of the children and reacts to them accordingly. Müller-Breckwoldt and Lipinski, p.158

Because of these intertwined consequences, I have come to believe in the course of my professional life working with children and adults with disabilities of all kinds, that these categories can help me to get a first impression of what may have been involved in the development of this particular person. It can also assist me to exchange information with other professionals. The categories may also help the person with the disability to identify him- or herself with a certain peer group. In a next step, however I must understand that for my work with a person with a disability, the diagnosis or the category provides nothing more than a tentative approach to get to know this person. It is inevitable, and also does more justice to the person we are working with, that we view these categories lightly and adopt a phenomenological way of looking at the entire person, together with this person, experiencing and describing every aspect of his or her personality—describing a very personal story.

Disability-Specific Developmental Factors

Working with clients who have a mental disability, there are times that I perceive empathy in the sense Shlien (1997, p. 73) writes, as an "act of attention, an effort", at other times it seems to be a natural attitude, a natural way of being present with the client. In any case I have found that in the work with mentally disabled clients this effort can be reinforced by understanding what implications the disability has had for the personal development of a client.

Children with disabilities, even more than other children, are confronted with conditions of worth. They will experience other people take over control of their lives, take decisions away from the child and know what is necessary and good for them. In the beginning this happens mostly because parents and caretakers believe there is some hope for improvement if they follow a tight schedule of therapies, guidelines and instructions. Most early interventions are focused on this negative aspect, on some lacking capacity, some deficiency, rather than on what capacities the child does have, as minor as they may appear to be. These children experience how part of them is not accepted, and they are liable to generalize this lack of acceptance to their entire personality.

Many of these therapies involve physical and psychological manipulations by others, and the children experience how their boundaries are constantly not being observed and respected, how their way of thinking and feeling is not being understood and respected. Eventually they themselves fail to develop adequate self-respect or awareness of their own needs, wishes and boundaries. They'll find other, even disturbing ways to influence and manipulate their environment, be it for example by rage attacks or by auto-mutilation. They learn not to take their feelings seriously and to exclude parts of their selves from their self-concept, when, for example, the parents avoid talking about the disability.

This process may continue throughout the child's entire life. Certain developmental aspects, such as sexuality for example, are considered not present in a teenager who has a mental disability. The development of an identity which is separate from the identity of the parents is also a difficult issue, in particular when these parents tend to overprotect their child, the child in a very real sense actually *being* dependent on them. In some cases I have observed parents, guided by their often disappointing experiences and their concern, deciding what their adult children will wear, interpreting what they are thinking, predicting what they will feel. In spite of their wish for the child to become as independent as possible, they do not realize that by acting thus they hamper their child's actualizing process.

When these children reach adulthood, many cannot take care of their own body. They need help washing or assistance toileting themselves. Sometimes, however, it is evident that they *could* have attended to these things, had their parents or caretakers considered it useful or possible to assist them in developing the skills. This can imply that the child did not have not opportunity to develop a sense of responsibility for his or her body and little sense of self-determination in that regard. As a result, people with disabilities may also not develop a sense of intimacy and shame leading to vulnerabilities to such dangers as sexual abuse. They may not learn to decide to what degree they want and need personal hygiene and how much they could do by themselves. They may not know definitely how to distinguish where the limits are to such hygienic measures and where it may or may not be appropriate to become sexually active. And even if they have acquired these capacities, they still need a certain amount of self-determination and courage to say yes or no.

In the field of child psychology we are confronted with many psychological theories on developmental psychology, which are partly based on physical capacities; here an interesting question arises: what happens when these capacities are not normally developed? Even though it might be helpful to wonder what impact the disability may have had on the child's personality development, none of these theories consider this at all. Mahler et al (1975) connect the mental birth of the individual with the detachment and individuation process which is necessary for the child to become an individual with an identity of his or her own. An important step in this individuation process is the rapprochement stage when the child starts to run away from his or her parents and come back again, apparently to reassure him- or herself and then run away again, discovering and conquering the world. I find this an interesting image, but I wonder what happens to the individuation when the child with paralysis never learns to run away. Or what about the effect of bowel and bladder incontinence, if learning to control these organs plays an important role in the development of autonomy? What happens to the child's discovery of sexuality when his or her genitals only seem to be a non-functional part of his or her body? All these questions cannot be answered here, but are meant to intensify the reader's awareness for the effect an impairment can have on personality development.

Although my clients are individuals with individual and unique problems and life issues, I have found that there is one thing that many of them seem to have in common: they seem to lack 'initiative' or 'creativity'. It is as if they never learned how to direct themselves, how to make decisions, how to solve problems. I wonder whether this is the result of a cognitive deficiency or rather reinforced as a secondary disability resulting from an over-protectionist attitude of primary care-takers in their early developmental years. Many parents are afraid something will happen to their children, and even more so their child lacks certain capacities! These parents often have difficulties in letting their child be confronted with and persevere through difficult situations. As a consequence their child does not learn to tolerate a certain level of frustration which may be an explanation for their tantrums, but the child also fails to develop creative ways in finding a solution or taking an initiative. Because of parents' anxiety as well as lack of the child's high self-concept the child does not dare to display initiative. If my hypothesis has merit and this lack of 'creativity' or 'initiative' is due to overprotection and anxiety, then the child actually has not received enough confirmation and affirmation.

The Person-Centered Approach

What for me makes the person-centered approach stand out specifically for the work with clients who have disabilities is the belief in the actualizing tendency, which leaves space for every possible development. Development, as Pörtner (1997) suggests, can be seen in every change, every adaptation a person has to perform in order to be able to live in a satisfactory way. These can be changes in "...their self-concept, their attitude and their habits...When we assume that the organism in principle is directed towards activating resources in order to be able to adapt itself to new life conditions, then it is not abstruse to trust that development is possible..." (p. 41). This can show itself in tiny little steps a person takes and which must be noticed and affirmed.

The person-centered approach does not expect clients to change in a specific direction. The therapist's or caretaker's *unconditional positive regard* and the *effort to understand a person in his or her internal frame of reference* allows the person to be whoever he or she is, to develop at whatever pace he or she chooses or is able to. *Congruence* will enable the therapist or caretaker to interact with the disabled client in an authentic and sincere way and to treat him or her respectfully. The presence of these core conditions increase the probability that the client can move in the direction of becoming his potential.

I think that at the base of the core conditions is unconditional positive regard. However, all three of these core conditions are parts of a whole attitude and are intertwined with each other, comparable with the steps of a dance. Here I will look more closely at the steps one by one. I will discuss empathy at the end not because I think it is the most or least important of the core conditions, but rather because I think it represents a huge challenge to try and understand a way of thinking or feeling or experiencing that may not be so different from our own but which is often expressed in a very different way and therefore can seem difficult to understand, and so I want to pay special attention to it.

The belief in the actualizing tendency

"Contrary to the views that see men's deepest instincts as destructive, I have found that when man is truly free to become what he most deeply is (as in the safe climate of therapy), when he is free to be his nature as a being capable of awareness, then he clearly moves towards wholeness and integration. (Rogers & Wood, 1974, p. 215)

Something that strongly attracted me to the person-centered approach was the concept of *the actualizing tendency*. It seemed to be the answer to a question I had been asking within myself for a long time. I only need to look at a child's way of moving around in the world to see that there is such a thing as this tendency for growth, and so many developmental factors can be understood in this context. A child growing up shows fear in certain situations; yet this same child is also driven by curiosity to explore the world. Both fear and curiosity are important for development, and in the best of cases, parents will offer safety or encourage the child according to his or her necessities and capacities. Eventually the child will learn to become autonomous. The three core conditions of the person-centered approach will facilitate this tendency towards personal growth in the most adequate way, because through the parents' empathy the child will learn to understand her own feelings, will accept them and will develop a self-concept in which her organismic experiences are integrated, i.e. become congruent. This process enables her to become an autonomous person.

This *actualizing tendency* is an axiom, it is a matter of believing or of one's view of the nature of human beings. Still, I believe evidence of it exists everywhere, and most people, professionals or not, seem to believe in it up to a limited extent. We expect a child at a certain point to start walking, to start communicating, to learn how to read and write. There is not much question about that. We make plans and have expectations for the child's future. These expectations and plans provide evidence of a usually unreflected upon belief in something like an actualizing tendency.

But when a child is born with a disability, professionals, and within a short time also the parents, often dismiss the actualizing tendency. Their way of interacting with this child can be dominated by the fact that the child is lacking certain capacities and that this has to be 'repaired' according to the values and the conditions of our society—practical conditions which present themselves in our every day life, but also conditions of worth on an inter- and intrapersonal level. And with this tendency to focus on what is missing, the lack of trust in the child's actualizing tendency includes the whole person of this child. If one missing part is focused upon, the whole gestalt is lost.

This child will grow up with a sense of being different and will experience this disability as a shortcoming. Of course a disability may lead to certain problems. It is not easy if I cannot hear well, as this may lead to my misunderstanding important concepts; a staircase is a problem if I am dependent on a wheelchair; and when my mental capacities are reduced I might not be able to learn how to read and write. The problem, however, is that the lack of the therapists' or parents' belief in the actualizing tendency leads to the child's development of a self-concept of being insufficient in every aspect. I have seen men and women with disabilities who often underestimate their own capacities. In some cases the denial of the disability may also lead to overestimation and efforts to be no different from other human beings who are not in some way physically or mentally impaired. And this attitude leads to a denial of certain aspects of their selves.

When years ago, I started to work with babies and toddlers with a large spectrum of disabilities, I also saw them as needy little persons whom I would have to teach a great deal or almost everything so they would 'grow'. I would enable them to compensate for their disabilities as far as possible. I was supposed to teach them how to grasp objects, how to look at the world, how to hear sounds, how to speak to me. But soon I found that I was pulling the grass to make it grow. Of course there were learnings with which they had great difficulties. What I began to learn for myself, however, was that when giving up my self-concept of being an expert, I learned important concepts from them: to "grasp" their way of experiencing, to look through their eyes, to listen to them more closely and to speak their language. Rogers said, "I find that one of the best, but most difficult ways for me to learn is to drop my own defensiveness, at least temporarily, and to try to understand the way in which this experience seems and feel to the other person" (1961, pp. 276-277). Changing my way of relating to these children and opening up for their way of experiencing provided ample evidence of the existence of the actualizing tendency.

I stopped seeing myself as the only 'teacher'. We began to be each others' teacher and pupil. I was able to approach them on a more equal level, as my importance was reduced and theirs was increased. I began to focus on the whole person and not only on the disability. This new focus changed my way of working with them and has paved the road for working in a person-centered way with adults with disabilities.

The Core Conditions

Unconditional positive regard

Working people who are mentally disabled, we are bound to be confronted with what is 'unknown', 'strange', 'alien' to us, and I believe that here lies a huge challenge to our ability in providing unconditional positive regard and full acceptance. This person may be alien to us and confusing, even frightening in his way of thinking, his way of expressing himself or in his behavior. His body may be distorted, spit maybe dribbling out of his mouth. He may be ugly to look at or difficult to understand in his speech. In general there is 'more' to accept than there usually is with people who do not have obvious disabilities.

If we succeed in accepting a person in her whole way of being, including everything there is within and about this person, then this opens up a vast space for the development of a relationship between the client and ourselves and consequently of the relationship the client has with himself.

In the lives of all of us, conditions of worth can be sensed everywhere, connected to every aspect of our way of being and living. While growing up children with disabilities come to experience these conditions of worth mostly in connection with their disability. They are not necessarily expressed in the sense of "I do not love you if you are like that", but rather it is intimated to them as "I so much wish you would not be the way you are." The most loving and caring parents have their ideas about how their child's happiness can be achieved, and to many people it seems that a disability is not the way to get there. These conditions of worth also exist more generally on a community level: the belief that people with a disability cannot live a satisfying and happy life is deeply rooted. The tendency to avoid even thinking about life with a disability is reflected in the fact that architects only recently have started to consider the necessities of a person with a physical disability entering and moving around in buildings and other public localities.

Let us first take the medical sector as another example: How often do future parents receive support in their wish to have their child, even after receiving the pre-genital diagnosis of a disability in this unborn baby? The more usual advice is the one to consider abortion, and often catastrophic possibilities are evoked in order to convince them that it is impossible to cope with this difficult situation.

These attitudes go further on a socio-economic level: Consider the expenses connected with the disability of this human being throughout his life. What is more, he is also not likely to ever contribute to the economy in the form of work or to pay taxes. In these times where part of our self-actualization and our self-esteem is attributed to our working activity and our income, it is difficult to imagine that we can draw self-esteem from ourselves also when we are capable of professionally activity. As a friend of mine put it once: "We are human *beings*, not human *doings*."

In school, integration has become an issue, and still it is realized only to a limited degree. A new standard has appeared called 'integrationability' to indicate up to what degree the child is able to adapt himself with his disability according to the needs of the environment. I do not believe that integration is achieved by adapting the environment entirely to the child's needs, as that would rather foster over-protection. The Latin word 'integration' means 'establishment (restoration) of a whole'. I believe that thinking about the interrelatedness between the community and the person with a disability, this wholeness is to be established in an equilibrium between the needs of that person and the given conditions of the society. That means that *both must be willing to adapt as much as possible to each other's needs, as is the case in any equal relationship between human beings.*

In this way such a relationship is not a matter of dependence, but one of interdependence. Even if a person is dependent on other people's assistance in many activities, he can be considered a whole person in his specific way of being. There is always autonomy and self-determination on an intrapsychic level, even if this outer dependency is present. When this person has learned to accept himself with his disability as part of his way of being a person, he can be autonomous in a different way than we usually think of, simply because he is respected by himself and by others as an individual. To achieve such self-respect is not easy for any of us, and even harder when relating to a person with a disability, as we live in this judgmental community. Yet it can be achieved if the parents and other important persons convey this unconditional attitude towards the disabled child. Then the child will be confronted with his boundaries, and they are closer than they are for a non-disabled child, and still he will not devaluate himself. This child will learn how to relate with these boundaries.

In order to facilitate this process, we must support the parents from the very beginning (see section about parents), and later we can convey this unconditionality to our clients ourselves through a person-centered attitude. This does not mean, according to my perception, that we act in a 'laissez-faire' manner. As I see, some of these clients need, at times, some guidance in the same way a child does. To a child it may be frightening to be in a new situation with a strange person in an unknown place. It could cause anxiety to not say anything and just wait until the child says or does something.

Recently I read a newspaper article saying that one important value in the society of this century, which was not at all a value in the last century or before, is *tolerance*. And even though prejudices are still very general, I think that we slowly are getting more and more used to differences. Even though it does not function always and everywhere in a satisfying way, integration of people with disabilities into society has become an issue, and being different is less prone to being stigmatized than it used to be. Children become more accustomed to being in class with children who have disabilities, and people with disabilities are increasingly standing up for their individual rights and their wish to be accepted the way they are.

Several times, at the end of a therapy process, clients have told me that one of the most important learnings in this relationship was to be "treated as an adult" and to be "taken seriously".

Congruence

Apart from the general necessity to be congruent, i.e. being aware of my feelings and emotions and distinguishing what is mine and what comes from the person I am working with, I believe it is necessary to know my own attitude towards disability in general and towards people with disabilities. For this I have to remember my own process of meaning-making regarding disability during my life, and do some self-exploring into how I feel about it today. Other issues in this context include 'weakness' or 'being different', 'needing help', 'being or feeling dependent', 'being an outsider', 'having a stigma'.

Still other issues that are helpful to consider are my own 'disability' or my own 'feeling disabled/incompetent/ powerless,' my 'being an outsider,' 'feeling stigmatized,' 'being dependent/helpless,' and my attitude towards these issues in relation to myself.

Thinking, for example, about my experiences with disability in my childhood, I felt surprise discovering that there *had* been two disabled children in my neighborhood: a boy who had quadriplegia, with splints on his lower legs and a strange posture; and a girl with Down's Syndrome whose sister went to the same school as I. I saw these children quite regularly on the street, but there was absolutely no contact whatsoever. They went to different schools and were picked up in special busses. I never asked the girl who went to school with me about her sister. Maybe I would have if she had been my friend. Whenever adults spoke about these children or children whit disabilities in general, they would use the term 'unhappy' or 'unlucky' children. At that time, this was a common expression for children with disabilities.

There was also a man in the village who could not speak. To us children he was frightening, but we also used him, to enrich our fantasy, as a fascinating, thrilling freak. Sometimes I had a slight understanding that behind his bawling speech there might be a normal human being whom I had no reason to be frightened of.

So, on the one hand I did not grow up with any close contact or experience with people with disabilities; the stage was set, however, for me to develop prejudices from early on. On the other hand, being an outsider myself for different reasons, I may have been able to develop an understanding of this way of being, and I still use the memory of this experience in order to understand how it may feel to be an outsider and not being accepted the way one is. An absolutely strong feeling of powerlessness and of fear, for example, may be involved. This awareness is extremely important for me, to know because I am aware that I have a tendency to 'coax' people with disabilities into standing up for themselves, instead of accepting each individual's rhythm. It is helpful to distinguish whether it is my anger-when I hear about bad treatment-or abuse, or whether I am resonating with my client.

For every person working in the social service field it is absolutely necessary to be vigilant about boundaries. To be aware of these boundaries and to act accordingly is the only way for preventing burn out. These boundaries may consist of not being able to work with a client who is drooling regularly, or of not wanting to work with several severely disabled clients on the same afternoon, which can be very tiring. These boundaries are individually different, and it is essential to recognize this difference.

Empathy

To begin with it is essential to distinguish between empathy and sympathy. As Shlien points out, Carl Rogers "wanted to avoid any tendency to pity, which he considered to be not kindness, but something approaching contempt" (1997, p. 70). The term 'unhappy children,' which I mentioned above, connotes pity, or judgmental sympathy, as it relates to a person with a disability.

Bozarth asserts that empathy primarily is "the way to communicate unconditional positive regard" (1998, p. 51) and that in the end, empathy and unconditional acceptance are the same experience. This way of being encountered or addressed is something many persons with disabilities have not experienced during their life, since they are often looked upon and treated with sympathy (or contempt—but is there a difference?) or treated as an 'object of education.' *To be accepted and understood in such an unconditional and empathic way is an entirely new experience for most of them.*

Here I would like to return to the developmental aspects with regard to empathy. Binder describes how the primary caretakers' "tendency to imitate and to comment on the behavior of the child is recognized as early empathic reflection, motor mimicry and affect attunement. These are considered to be primitive forms of communicative empathy" (1998, p. 221). A child learns to name and understand feelings through the reflection of the primary caretaker. In the beginning this process occurs through imitation of the faces the child makes, the words the child speaks. Later the interactions based on empathy become more differentiated. With respect to this Binder mentions "arousing interest, sharing attention, cheering up and distracting, soothing and offering help," a kind of empathy essential for the social/emotional development of the self, even before a self-concept is established.

Children with mental disabilities may have a different form of emotional expression, and therefore their parents may have difficulties in understanding them. Example of this are: an autistic child who shows minimal facial expression or doesn't admit eye contact; a child who cries day and night without obvious reason; a child who does not develop speech. Empathic reflection can become extremely difficult for the parents of these children. This difficulty may lead to a deficient development of the child's empathic ability which is connected with "deficiencies in the regulation of emotions, in the capacity for spontaneous social behavior, in social competence and in the capacity for emotional self-expression. There is also a lack of self-confidence…and of self- and environmental control" (Binder, 1998, p. 224).

What Binder describes for persons with schizophrenia, in many ways also is valid for persons with a mental disability. They may struggle with understanding and regulating their own feelings which, in times of stress can lead to emotional outbursts, intense states of anxiety, tantrums and insecurity. Their self-concept in many cases is a reflection of the image their parents or society has conveyed to them. Their experienced incompetence and powerlessness to control their environment in a healthy way can lead to a continuous effort to manipulate this environment, for example by such responses as tantrums, expressions of helplessness or even by automutilative behavior.

A client of mine who is quadriplegic and therefore not only has little control over the muscles of his arms and legs, but also of his mouth, tried to hurt himself with a pair of scissors after the bus driver told him that "they should have given him a shot to calm him down" when he had shown his anger about this person for being always late. My own anger and feeling of utmost powerlessness were a reflection of how he was feeling. His muscles did not enable him to hit this person, his mouth gave him no opportunity to express spontaneously what he felt. His rage turned inside and made him grab these scissors to find a valve for expressing his experience. I remained present with him in this feeling of powerless rage, an emotional state which was not the first such experience in his life. His parents had often threatened to place him in a psychiatric ward.

As this client's speech was not always easy to understand, especially in the beginning, I reflected each word I understood in the same way as is done in a Word-by-Word-Reflection in pre-therapy (which I will elaborate upon below); in this way he was able to hear what I had understood and what was necessary for him to correct. He developed incredibly creative ways of making himself understood; I too had to be creative in my thinking. Though sometimes I struggled to make sense of his words, only seldom was it necessary to give up. At those times we often joked about *my* 'disability,' that is, *my* limited capacity to understand.

My empathic understanding slowly made it possible for him to turn the rage towards this man whose words had been so degrading and aggressive and towards the company who hired him. He also started to understand that people without disabilities also sometimes feel absolutely powerless. He ended up working in a self-help group of people with disabilities who tried to get politicians to create a position for an ombudsman for complaints of citizens with disabilities; he also gave me a scarf he had painted of a person in a wheelchair like himself and a walking person like me, on which he had written "who can walk is disabled". Apart from succeeding in regulating his own emotions more adequately, he had also developed a personal relationship with me, which in the beginning he was not able to relate to me adequately. I was nothing other than a Wailing Wall.

"Empathic processes and their successful realization in understanding, communication and action lead…to increased well-being and self-esteem" (Binder, 1998, p. 218). "The outcomes of therapy include the client becoming…(3.) more effective in problem solving; this suggests more enhanced psychological adjustment, increased degree of positive self-regard, more acceptance of others, and behavior being perceived as more social and mature by others." (Bozarth, 1998, p. 44) Even if these outcomes may seem to lead toward too high expectations in the case of clients who have a mental disability, I assert that they are valid. Even though people with disabilities may never be able to be completely self-responsible due to their impairment, their self can be subject to changes and development in the release of the actualizing tendency. A 24-year old slightly mentally retarded woman who was my client very quickly picked up my unconditional acceptance and empathy for her, often also telling me in an admiring tone: "You really do understand what I am talking about, don't you?" And even though in the end, whenever I was in the institution where she works, she would present me to her colleagues proudly calling me "*my* psychologist!" She developed some self-responsibility adequate to her level of cognitive development and decided herself at a certain point that therapy had been enough and that she might come back to work on another issue later when she would feel it was the right time.

Often the issue these clients bring to therapy are related to difficulties with parents when they leave home to live in a living community for people with disabilities. The parents have problems in letting go and the clients introject their parents' anxiety and feel torn between their insecurity about their need to move away form the security of their parents on the one hand and their wish to become more independent and develop a life of their own. Here the affirmation and confirmation they receive through unconditional positive regard and empathic understanding helps them to find security *within themselves*, at least to give it a try, or to decide to stay for some more time with their parents. Whatever the course of action, it is important that it is *their* decision.

Until now I have been using examples of clients who are mildly mentally disabled, who are still able to verbalize their thoughts and feelings, although sometimes on a rather basic level and who definitely are able to establish and to maintain psychological contact with me. There are also, however, clients whose way of expressing themselves is much more limited or sometimes resembles a psychotic way of expression. Some have no ability to speak.

Generally empathy with clients who are mentally disabled can be essentially the same as with other clients. The ability of the client to communicate verbally plays a role here. Many professionals claim that the client has to be able to express him- or herself verbally for the therapist to be able to be empathic. This claim is a myth.

On the side of the therapist, empathy "is often wordless." It "operates on data such as smell, sight, and sound" (Shlien, 1997, p. 77). In working with clients who are unable to express themselves so clearly, the use of *my* senses, in order to develop empathic understanding, becomes more essential. This activity (or process) can actually be an intended effort as mentioned above. I strive to open up every element of my organism which can contribute to this process of understanding the other person's frame of reference. I have sometimes called this for myself *organismic empathy*.

From my client's perspective my empathic effort may be conveyed by words, but also by the expression of my eyes, my posture, my gestures. With clients who are more severely retarded, I have to work on a very concrete level in the here and now. Here Prouty's pre-therapy has shown itself to be helpful. His procedure was developed in order to work with patients who are schizophrenic and mentally retarded psychiatric who were not in psychological contact with the therapist or caretaker. I have come to see it as a deep form of empathy, which has led to clear manifestations of self-actualization in these clients.

Prouty (1994) developed five different categories of reflections which help the client get in contact with themselves and their environment within time and space. These reflections remind me of the way mothers and fathers continuously comment about what their babies and toddlers are doing, thus helping them to develop an understanding of themselves and the objects or persons around them. Parents do this, seemingly instinctively, in the preverbal phase and in the beginning of the verbal phase of their child's development. The clients to whom I am referring here seem to be in comparable developmental stages, although it is not always certain whether they can develop any further. But even if they do not, it has been evident that their life quality was improved as they felt understood by their caretakers who applied pre-therapy. I have seen a young woman who never would look anybody directly in their eyes, who merely sat with her head hanging down, mumbling to herself. Her caretaker started to work in a pre-therapeutic way with her in individual sessions. After some sessions there was a moment where her caretaker repeated in a Word-by-Word-Reflection what she had understood, and as she had misunderstood something, the woman suddenly looked up, straight into her caretaker's eyes and repeated persistently what she wanted her to understand. Subsequently there were more and more moments of real psychological contact. Ultimately she was considered for psychotherapy.

In supervision with caretakers, we worked on practical ways to improve their empathic capacities by enhancing their range of experiences: driving a wheelchair or walking around the house blindfolded for a weekend opens up whole new perspectives. It can become a new kind of experiencing oneself in an unknown and difficult situation. I learned how it feels to be so dependent on someone to push me or lead me around, sometimes even without asking me if I am actually in need of assistance. A caretaker shared an interesting dream about being deaf and blind, and after this simulated activity, she managed to more deeply understand her client, who was both deaf and blind, when he had his 'psychotic' outbursts.

I would like to mention one last aspect which needs empathic understanding by the therapist: clients with a mental disability also ask questions much more frequently than other clients. Bozarth states, "…the therapist should be inclined to address client's questions by being genuine and open to honoring their requests, as well as offering empathic responses to verify the therapist's experiences of empathic understanding during the interaction process" (1997, p. 93). With clients who have mental disabilities I have often found their questions to be expressive of a need for affirmation and for anxiety reduction. At times it is important to merely understand these dynamics; at other times, specifically in the beginning of the therapeutic process, answering the question can provide evidence of understanding this need of the client in the immediate moment and eventually contribute to the basic trust which is necessary for a therapeutic relationship.

Outcome

People may think that the expression "fully functioning person" which Rogers used to describe the (ideal) outcome of client-centered psychotherapy is somewhat ironic in this context: How can a person become fully functioning when his or her functions are impaired on one or many levels without the possibility of "repair"?

Still, such a model is merely an ideal which shows a direction for personal development. Evidently functional impairment of any kind reduces the level of 'fully functioning' for the person who has a disability. As a client-centered therapist does not judge the person or compare him or her to others with or without a disability, but only pays attention to the person's specific way of being, he or she strives for maximum functioning *for that person*. What makes client-centered so effective in this context is the fact that Rogers has striven to consider the unique individual, and decries normative considerations.

When a child, for example, has a sensory impairment and therefore will probably never learn to communicate fully as hearing people do, it is a great achievement when he or she begins to speak words, and even if that child is already six years old when this happens or if it is clear that speech may be limited to little more than ten or twenty words it is indeed a great achievement. Parents and caretakers often develop an acute awareness for and appreciation of these small signs of progress.

In this sense the outcome of psychotherapy can be considerable for these clients: their self-awareness and self-esteem can be enhanced; their self-determination can be reinforced; their self-security can become stronger and thus, their independence can be developed further; their life-quality can be improved.

All these outcomes are achievements to hope for, but in the beginning of therapy it is not sure whether these are the client's goals and there is no way to say whether such outcomes will be achieved. Again and again, however, I have been surprised with how fruitful these processes developed. I am absolutely sure that the three core conditions are the foundations for these outcomes, but only when the therapist holds a solid belief in the actualizing tendency. Even though I know that I (too) often have clear ideas about what a good outcome could be, Jerold Bozarth has described it very well with the following words: "If the individual can be affirmed in being who he or she is at the moment then that is good enough" (1998, p. 49).

Parents of disabled children

When I begin working with clients who are mentally disabled, they come with an entire history of their developing self, self-concept, behaviors and ways of relating to themselves and to their environment.

As I have indicated above it would be extremely important to start at the beginning, i.e. at the point where the disability is communicated to the parents or when the child and his or her parents are very much at the beginning of their story, in order to support a positive development. Therefore I want to offer a short overview of how the person-centered approach could be helpful to these families.

The parents are the ones who accompany and guide this child through life: They are the ones who must give up their conventional ideas and hopes about the development of their child. The birth of a child with a disability is the beginning of a story about a relationship, and it is essential to help them ultimately to perceive this loss as more than a sad story, but rather as a story which can include highlights or happiness.

It happens too often that the message is communicated to the parents by a member of the medical staff who merely wants to get it over with. The message often is abruptly given in passing or at the bedside of the child. Frequently it is just one person who is informed: the father because the mother is still in the clinic where the child was born; the mother because she is the one who went to see the doctor because she thought something was wrong. Whoever it is, that person does not only have to cope with his or her difficult emotions after hearing such terrible news, but also has the heavy task of communicating the message to his or her partner. I plea for a procedure where both parents are informed, whenever possible, even if this means that the doctor would have to go to the clinic where the mother is.

Communicating a disability to the parents is not only a matter of communicating the diagnosis and the perspectives. It is also about facilitating the development of a loving relationship between the parents and the child. And after this there should be some psychological assistance or guidance, especially because the shock is so overwhelming that, too often, the parents remember only the diagnosis and the atmosphere of the conversation. The medical staff must be prepared to repeat the facts again and again, patiently, until they are integrated in the parents' awareness, in their understanding and experiencing, in their lives. It is necessary to have some knowledge about common emotional responses aspects that may influence the impact the message has on these parents.

I would like to offer some examples of situations likely to play a role in the individual reaction of a parent who hears such news.

Generally the parents' relationship to this child does not start at birth, but much earlier, i.e. during pregnancy, in the family tradition, in the mind of the parents to be, of the grandparents and of the siblings. Their idea of the child that is going to be born is, of course, a construction, an image of a hoped for child. And that image shatters to pieces. The parents are faced with reconstructing their image of the child, and they must do this in a much more radical way than other parents. This means that they have to integrate this 'new' child into their awareness. They do this each at his or her own rhythm. Some parents resist this process for a long time; they will continue to 'see' a healthy child for a while and fight against the new reality within themselves.

This integration may also be influenced by some unique factors related to the personality of the parents, to their previous experiences with disabilities, their life projects, the gender of the baby, the presence of other siblings, the reactions of their environment, their financial situation and also to the degree and the origin of the disability.

In order to achieve a positive integration, parents often go through a process involving several kinds of emotions which are comparable with the stages of grief described by Elisabeth Kübler-Ross for people who have experienced a loss or who learn that they will die. It can be just as painful to lose an imagined healthy child as a real child. The difference lies in the fact that the child does not die, and the process may reach the stage of integration, but it may repeat itself—possibly in a milder form—at each new phase in the life of the child: when he or she starts going to kindergarten and to school and the difference between their child and other children becomes more evident; when other children begin going out with friends, and begin to date; when these other children start to work; when these other children, by now adults, marry and have children.

These emotional reactions do not always take place in the same order nor are they necessarily experienced by everyone. These reactions often include incredibility and negation, an effort to keep this reality out of their awareness, an effort for self-protection; feelings of guilt or accusations, an effort to find a way to explain how this could happen and to thus get it under control, at least on a cognitive level; rage at the medical staff, at the partner, an effort to fight against a feeling of powerlessness; grief, sadness—as long as it doesn't result in a depression—all these experiences can bring the person closer to acceptance and integration of the fact that life has changed in a radical way. Only then is there a possibility that the parents will arrive at accepting their child as different, even feel pride when he or she makes progress, as tiny as their child may be. Here the story of this child and its parents can begin to take a positive turn for them all, a story of relating and mutual learning, of enriching each other.

In this beginning stage and throughout the further life of the child, the problems its parents are confronted with can range form self-doubt, rejection of the child, strain and exhaustion, anxiety, education issues, maltreatment etc.; in a later phase of life, the issues of letting go and of sexuality become paramount. While supporting these parents from the very beginning and at any other stage of life, it is helpful to accompany them in this process and accept whatever emotional state they are in. Each stage is a step towards acceptance, and therefore necessary to be achieved. When their feelings and thoughts are acknowledged, respected, and taken seriously, when they are not treated as incompetent or poor parents, they may be able to develop a sense of competence in their role as parents. By being accepted in their anger and sadness, in their vulnerability and doubts, they will move towards accepting themselves with these feelings, and not experience them solely as weakness. And in the end they may be able to accept the "weakness" of their child as part of its being, instead of regarding it as a taint. They will feel affirmed and confirmed, and thus regain confidence in themselves; as a consequence they will communicate this confidence also to the child.

Empathic understanding will help parents to understand their own feelings and consequently to accept them as part of themselves. Congruence is necessary for the person working with these parents in order to be non-defensive and open for whatever comes from them. This way parents can learn to be accepting, empathic and congruent with themselves and consequently with their children, thus supporting them in their development of a positive self-concept and self-competence, of a capacity for emotional self-regulation and of relating to their environment, all within their individual boundaries and possibilities.

Elisabeth Zinschitz lives in Vienna, Austria. She holds a degree in languages, studies psychology and completed a six year training program in client-centered psychotherapy. She has a private practice where she offers psychotherapy for clients who are disabled and non-disabled; Further she offers supervision for caretakers as well as counseling for parents of persons with disabilities. She has three children, one of whom has a physical disability (spina bifida). Before becoming a psychotherapist she worked in early care with children who have disabilities and their families.

References

Binder, U. (1998). Empathy and empathy development with psychotic clients. In B. Thorne & E. Lambers (Eds.), **Person-centred therapy. A European perspective** (pp. 216-230). London: Sage.

Bozarth, J. (1997). Empathy from the framework of client-centered theory and the Rogerian hypothesis. In A. C. Bohart & L. S. Greenberg (Eds.), **Empathy reconsidered: New directions in psychotherapy** (pp. 81-102). Washington: American Psychological Society.

Bozarth, J. (1998). **Person-centred therapy: A revolutionary paradigm.** Ross-on-Wye: PCCS Books.

Feuser, G. (1996). Testimony before the Austrian parliament on October 29 in a hearing about the integration of disabled children in regular schools. Vienna, Austria.

Küböer-Ross, E. (1969). **On death and dying.** New York, London: The MacMillan Company—Collier Macmillan Ltd.

Mahler, M. S., Pine, F., & Bergmann, A. (1975). **The psychological birth of the human infant.** New York: Basic Books.

Müller-Breckwoldt, H., & Lipinski, C. (1988). "Im Traum, da kann ich laufen!"—Die Körperbehinderung Spina bifida im Erleben von Kindern an der Schwelle zur Pubertät. Ein Beispiel personenzentrierter Gruppenarbeit in der Rehabilitation. In U. Esser & K. Sander (Eds.), Personenzentrierte Gruppentherapie: Therapeutischer Umgang mit der Person und mit der Gruppe. Heidelberg.

Peters, H. (1992). **Psychotherapie bij geestelijk gehandicapten.** Amsterdam: Swets & Zeitlinger.

Pörtner, M. (1996). **Ernstnehmen—Zutrauen—Verstehen. Personzentrierte Haltung im Umgang mit geistig behinderten und pflegebedürftigen Menschen.** Stutgart: Klett-Cotta.

Prouty, G. F. (1990). Pre-therapy: A theoretical evolution in the person-centered/experiential psychotherapy of schizophrenia and retardation.

In G. Lietaer, J. Rombauts, & R van Balen (Eds.), **Client-centered and experiential psychotherapy in the nineties.** Leuven: Leuven University Press. (pp. 645-658) .

Prouty, G. F. (1994). **Theoretical evolutions in person-centered/experiential therapy: Applications to schizophrenic and retarded psychoses.** Westport: Praeger Publishers.

Rogers, C. R. (1951). **Client-centered psychotherapy.** Boston: Houghton Mifflin.

Rogers, C. R. (1961). **On becoming a person.** Boston: Houghton Mifflin.

Rogers, C. R., Wood, J. K. (1974). **Client-centered theory.** In A. Burton (Ed.), Operational Theories of Personality. New York: Brunner-Mazel. pp. 212-258.

Shlien, J. (1997). Empathy in psychotherapy: A vital mechanism? Yes. Therapist's conceit? All too often. By itself enough? No. In A. C. Bohart & L. S. Greenberg (Eds.), **empathy reconsidered: New directions in psychotherapy** (pp 63-80). Washington: American Psychological Society.

Thorne, B. (1992). **Carl Rogers.** London: Sage.

Zinschitz, E. (1998). The person-centred approach in work with disabled persons. **Counselling: The Journal of the British Association for Counselling,** 9(3).

Zinschitz, E. (in press). L'annonce d'un handicap—le début d'une histoire: "Pourque le blé puisse croitre, il faut d'abord cultiver le champs." In G. Zribi & J. Sarfaty (Eds.), **Construction de soi et handicap mental: L'enfant et l'adulte handicapé mental dans leur environnement familial, social et institutionel.** Paris: Editions de l'Ecole Nationale de la Santé Publique.

Implications of the Person-centered Approach for Pastoral Counseling

Doug Bower

When I started two similar research projects (Bower, 1985, 1989), I could not find one pastoral counselor who qualified for those studies. I asked pastoral counselors who were familiar with the literature to recommend prominent person-centered colleagues, but they could produce no names even of a lesser-known colleague who claimed adherence to the person-centered approach. I had met many who are familiar with the literature and even use the core conditions in some way, but none that called themselves person-centered pastoral counselors. Since then I have met and interacted with three besides myself.

This difficulty was unexpected, as Rogers is acknowledged as having a great deal of influence on the pastoral counseling movement in the fifties and sixties. His articles appeared in The Journal of Pastoral Care and Pastoral Psychology. His books were mandatory reading in seminaries and clinical programs. He was referred to by leaders in pastoral counseling and pastoral theological literature. Yet no person-centered pastoral counselor could be found.

I was taught that Seward Hiltner, Thomas C. Oden, Carroll A. Wise and Don S. Browning were influenced greatly by Rogers. However, neither Wise nor Browning appears to maintain Rogerian concepts. I have found only Oden, a pastoral theologian, to be a strong adherent to Rogers' views. Hiltner articulated an adequate definition of empathy, but he stopped short of addressing the process of being empathic. Browning notes that Hiltner's notion of "eductive counseling" is similar to Rogers' nondirective approach. Yet, the definition of "eductive counseling," implying the process of drawing out is quite dissimilar from the definition of empathy, which describes the process of entering into. Hiltner's "eductive counseling" is aimed at getting the client to do something, while Rogers' empathy is aimed at the only goal of the therapist, to enter into and perceive the world of the client as the client sees it, the client doesn't have to do anything at all except be himself.

I return to this issue after 11 years not having changed my mind about person-centered pastoral counselors. I still only know a handful who call themselves person-centered. Yet, I will acknowledge my experience is limited to the Atlanta—Athens area, the Association for the Advancement of the Person-Centered Approach, the American Psychotherapy Association, and as a supervisor of graduate students at Ft. Valley State.

My hopes are to reexpand my professional world by rejoining the American Counseling Association and thus increase the possibility of meeting other pastoral counselors who call themselves person-centered. Yet, I am skeptical of finding many. I didn't when I was a member in other organizations and I really don't expect that has changed.

I mainly return to this subject of person-centered pastoral counseling because that is where my heart is. I am a pastor, pastoral counselor. My faith rests in the life, death, and resurrection of Jesus Christ. I am quite fundamental about that. I have found that I believe the person-centered approach is the best way for me to honor the concept "And just as you want people to treat you, treat them in the same way" Luke 6:31 [New American Standard Bible], and to honor Jesus' comment "'Come to Me, all who are weary and heavy-laden, and I will give you rest. 'Take My yoke upon you, and learn from Me, for I am gentle and humble in heart; and you shall find rest for your souls. 'For My yoke is easy, and My load is light'" Matthew 11:28-30 [NASB]. In short, I haven't found anything more pastoral than offering people empathy, acceptance, and genuineness.

What happened?

It is clear there has been a courtship with Rogers, but there was never a marriage. Some pastoral counseling theorists may have gone to bed with Rogerian theory, but there has never been a commitment to that theory. It appears that there has never been an assimilation of the theory to the point that a larger percentage of pastoral counselors claimed they were person-centered. Pastoral counselors have adopted psychoanalytic, TA, Gestalt and other theories. Yet, although many have come to acknowledge Rogers' thought as significant, I have seen few person-centered pastoral counseling practitioners.

Rogers was regarded as having tremendous potential for pastoral care and counseling. According to Robert C. Fuller (1984), Rogers' nondirective approach offered ready assimilation in comparison with other approaches examined in pastoral counseling. "Client-centered therapy requires less formal training than other psychotherapeutic models.... It can, therefore, be more easily introduced to seminary students and even full-time ministers whose schedules do not permit extensive psychological training" (p. 356).

On the surface, this claim would appear to be true. However, being empathic is not as easy as it appears, nor is understanding Rogers' concept of genuineness. How does one know when one is empathic? What does it mean to be congruent? Further, exercising acceptance and unconditional positive regard can be difficult. While I still use the term "unconditional positive regard," I no longer see it as unconditional. All of the core conditions require as intense a degree of interaction with Rogerian theory as practicing psychoanalysis does with Freudian theory. Regarding a superficial understanding of Rogers, (Bozarth and Mitchell, 1981) comment that

students and practitioners who believe that they are practicing the Client-Centered Approach...often have not learned the essence of this therapeutic effort. They are familiar with "reflection" and the with the importance of "developing a relationship." Too often, however, they equate the Client-Centered Approach to Human Relations Training Models. They view Client-Centered Therapy as only a prerequisite to other kinds of responding and miss the entire essence of the approach.

Further, Fuller (1984) states that Rogers is easy to assimilate because the jargon is simple. "Rogers's writings employ less jargon and are thus more accessible to a general reading knowledge" (p. 356). He apparently feels Rogers is easily understood. However, there is a great deal of depth in Rogers' thinking that is frequently overlooked. He is often misread and his readers may often take it for granted that they understand the approach. Fuller himself admits this: "I would even go so far as to state that the vast majority of theologians who have studied Rogers's works have either misread or distorted the fundamental character of what might be labeled the broadly religious and spiritual thrust of his psychological writings" (p. 363). After spending over 18 years grappling with Rogers' theory, I would go on to say there has been a significant failure to accept even the psychological aspects of his writings, despite the acknowledgment of the impact of Rogers in the psychotherapeutic field.

Where does the tension rest?

The most obvious tension lies in what is viewed as the limitations of the approach. The conditions of empathy, acceptance and congruence may be regarded as necessary but not sufficient for growth. This is exemplified by Clinebell (1966), who adds the missing ingredients which he believes can complete the necessary and sufficient conditions:

The Rogerian method provides a firm foundation but not the entire edifice of an adequate approach to counseling....The Rogerian model has tended to make the minister feel that he should strenuously avoid the use of his authority....In contrast, the revised model (which I propose) is based on the conviction that it is often constructive, even essential, for the pastor to use his authority selectively in sustaining, guiding, feeding (emotionally, inspiring, confronting, teaching and encouraging persons to function responsibly. (pp. 30-31)

Another tension lies in a pessimistic skepticism about the human condition, rooted traditionally on the theological influence of Paul, Augustine, Martin Luther, John Calvin and others. Mankind is made up of sinners who are incapable of doing good apart from the grace of God. Left to their own devices, mankind will continue to kill and maim fellow human beings. Left to their own devices, human beings will be destructive; they cannot be trusted:

Beware the beast man, for he is the devil's pawn. Alone among God's primates, he kills for sport or lust or greed. Yea, he will murder his brother to possess his brother's land. Let him not breed in great numbers for he will make a desert of his home and yours. Shun him, for he is the harbinger of death. (Serling & Wilson, quote from film)

Another tension rests in the perception of the authority of the pastor. Apparently, some pastoral counselors and pastoral theologians have felt this authority is threatened when the person-centered approach is adopted.

The pastoral counselor, in adopting the strategies of client-centered therapy, risked blurring his or her distinct identity as a representative of the Christian church....

The exclusive use of client-centered or "eductive" counseling techniques would, for example, appear to be a complete abdication of responsibility for confronting persons with the demands of moral and spiritual existence....A further concern...is that nondirective approaches to pastoral care and guidance ultimately lead to the impoverishment of the sacramental, mystical, and contemplative elements of Christian spirituality. The utterly optimistic view of human nature upon which Rogers' theory rests is...inconducive to fostering attitudes that orient individuals to look beyond themselves in their search for meaningful existence. (Fuller, 1984, pp. 359-360)

I believe that these criticisms slip into two categories. The first is a failure to accept the optimistic view of human nature. Rogers' theory is regarded as naive. This criticism fails to note Rogers' awareness of the difficulty and even the terror of the human situation.

I would not want to be misunderstood on this. I do not have a Pollyanna view of human nature. I am quite aware that out of defensiveness and inner fear individuals can and do behave in ways which are incredibly cruel, horribly destructive, immature, regressive, anti-social, hurtful. Yet one of the most refreshing and invigorating parts of my experience is to work with such individuals and to discover the strongly positive directional tendencies which exist in them, as in all of us, at the deepest levels. (Rogers, 1961, p. 27)

The second criticism concerns the exercise of authority. Rogers was not anti-authority; he was anti-authoritarian. He did not believe in controlling others. Domination by confrontation, direction, and pointing out discrepancies in behavior are manifestations of an authoritarian, "I am the expert" attitude. A vein of such authoritarianism runs through the history of the church and its clergy. What Rogers was interested in is personal power. One gains authority in the person-centered approach by being able to give up institutional authority and by recognizing and accepting the personal power of other persons. (Bozarth, 1985, 1998)

A new paradigm for pastoral counseling

The person-centered approach has more to offer than human relationship training. It addresses an inner dimension of being. I have seen little in the pastoral literature which is similar to Rogers' approach even though many claim to have been influenced by his thinking (Browning, 1976; Faber & van der Schoot, 1962; Gerkin, 1984; Hiltner, 1958; Oates, 1974; Oden, 1978; Patton, 1983). Of these, I consider only Oden person-centered based on what I read, but have some room to consider Browning person-centered. The others make no claims to being person-centered though they are clearly familiar with the person-centered approach. The secular literature is similar. "The concepts which are the crux of the person-centered approach and which reflect the very essence of a 'new age paradigm' have been secondarily considered and barely mentioned in the literature" (Bozarth, 1985, p. 6).

Potentials of the person-centered approach for pastoral counseling

The person-centered approach offers several principles of potential value to pastoral counseling. The first of these principles is that the presupposition of the process of the actualizing and formative tendencies—on the individual and the universal level—is the very foundation of the person-centered approach. "Rogers is explicit that the actualizing tendency, which is a characteristic of organic life; and the formative tendency, which is a characteristic of the universe as a whole '...are the foundation blocks of the person centered approach' (Rogers, 1980)" (Bozarth, 1985, p. 7.)

The person-centered pastoral counselor would have a trust and faith in the self-actualizing capacity of the client. "Practice, theory, and research make it clear that the person-centered approach rests on a basic trust in human beings, and in all organisms" (Rogers, 1961, p. 117). "The therapist must be able to act on the belief that the individual will move in the direction of self actualization when the therapist creates an atmosphere of acceptance and attends to the concrete-experiential flow of the client" (Bozarth, & Mitchell, 1981, p. 2).

Such an attitude is pivotal to the person-centered approach: "The fact is that if therapists are not able to act on this belief then they are not practicing Client-Centered Therapy....It is essential that therapists have nearly unfaltering 'faith' that individuals, given the opportunity, will engage in an optimal mode of experiencing" (Bozarth & Mitchell, p. 4).

The second principle is that the locus of control lies with the client. Can the client be him or herself in the presence of the therapist? Can the therapist recognize the client's inner ability to move in a self directive way?

Therapists often have difficulty being with their clients when the clients are 'muddled' or do not clearly communicate expected progress as perceived by the therapist. At the same time, therapist often seems patently unwilling to 'allow' the client to be extremely sad or in pain or psychotic. Their misperception…in therapy is primarily the view the relationship can be developed in such a way that the therapist can then guide the client towards appropriate direction and action. Focusing on the therapist's authoritative expertise often becomes more important than creating the atmosphere which allows the client to achieve self-direction.

Many therapists assume that their competence and progress is judged relative to how able they are to motivate clients to address and resolve problems in living. Thus the client is viewed in terms of what "ought to be discussed" or "what the person should do" (i.e. in terms of the therapist as authoritative expert)….(Bozarth & Mitchell, pp, 3-4)

In the person-centered approach the emphasis is not on how astutely the counselor can predict or interpret behavior (Rogers, 1977). The emphasis is on giving up the position of the power of the "expert" in order to become empathic (Bozarth, 1985, 1999). There is a "willingness of the facilitator to give up institution 'position power' for the opportunity to have personal influence, interaction…(Bozarth, 1981, p. 119).

In relationship to the locus of control, the pastoral counselor in the person-centered approach does not presuppose anything about the direction of the client's progress. That is, the pastoral counselor does not presuppose how the client can "get better." The pastoral counselor accepts the client in his own "idiosyncratic way by only assuming the self-actualized tendency without presupposing what the client should do, or become, or be during or beyond the psychotherapeutic encounter" (Bozarth, 1985, p. 1).

The last principle pertinent to pastoral counseling is that the role of the pastoral counselor is that of having certain attitudinal principles or qualities: empathy, acceptance and congruence.

To be true to the person-centered approach is to maintain a way of being, based on attitudes instead of techniques.

The therapist's role in the person-centered approach can be simply stated: Be real (genuine); be nonjudgmentally caring (unconditional positive regard); and enter the world of the client as if you are the client (empathy). Having these attitudinal qualities, the therapist 1) does not presuppose what a client might do, be, or become; and 2) has only one intention, i.e., to enter the world of the other "as if" he/she is the person. It is by the therapist being a person who has these characteristics that the client perceives the characteristics and personal growth is promoted....(Bozarth, 1985, p. 10)

Summary

The person-centered approach has ostensibly had an influence on the pastoral counseling movement. However, it has often been misread, rejected or superficially understood. In as much as there are few significant leaders in the pastoral counseling arena which are Rogerian, the person-centered approach has not been assimilated.

Rogers offers pastoral counseling a new paradigm: 1) to trust and have faith in the capacity of the human being to move in a self directive way, 2) to give up the position of institutional authority and expertise and allow the locus of control to rest with the client, and 3) to maintain the attitudinal principles of empathy, acceptance and congruence (genuineness).

Bower, D. W. (1985). Assumptions and attitudes of the Rogerian person-centered approach to counseling: Implications for pastoral counseling. Unpublished research project, Columbia Theological Seminary, Atlanta, Ga.

Bower, D. W. (1989). The attributes of five person-centered therapists. Unpublished doctoral dissertation, University of Georgia, Athens, Ga.

Bozarth, J. D. (1981). **The Person-centered approach in the large community group**. In G.Gazda (Ed.), **Innovations to group psychotherapy**. Springfield: Charles C. Thomas.

Bozarth, J. D. (1985). Quantum theory and the Person-centered approach. **Journal of Counseling and Development**, 64(3), 179-182.

Bozarth, J. D. (1998). **Person-centered therapy: A revolutionary paradigm**. Ross-on-Wye: PCCS Books.

Bozarth, J. D., & Mitchell, S. (1981). Functional Dimensions of the Person-Centered Approach in Therapy. Unpublished paper.

Browning, D. S. (1976). **The moral context of pastoral care**. Philadelphia: Westminster Press.

Clinebell, Jr., H. J. (1966). **Basic types of pastoral counseling**. Nashville: Abingdon.

Faber, H., & Van der Schoot, E. (1962). **The art of pastoral conversation: Effective counseling through personal encounter**. Nashville: Abington.

Fuller, R. C. (1984). Rogers's impact on pastoral counseling and contemporary religious reflection," in R. E. Levant & J. M. Shlien (Eds.), **Client-centered therapy and the person-centered approach** (pp. 352-369). New York: Praeger.

Gerkin, C. V. (1984). **The living human document: Re-visioning pastoral counseling in a hermeneutical mode**. Nashville: Abingdon.

Hiltner, S. (1958). **Preface to pastoral counseling**. Nashville: Abingdon.

Jackson. E. N. (1983). **Parish counseling**. New York: Jason Aronson.

Oates, W. E. (1974). **Pastoral counseling**. Philadelphia: Westminster Press.

Oden, T. C. (1978). **Kerygma and counseling**. New York: Harpers.

Patton, J. (1983). **Pastoral counseling: A ministry of the church**. Nashville: Abingdon.

Rogers, C. R. (1961). **On becoming a person**. Boston: Houghton Mifflin.

Rogers, C. R. (1977). **On personal power**. New York: Delta.

Back to the Very Basic Basics

Self-actualization: The Foundation of the Person-Centered Approach

Doug Bower

The concept of self-actualization is an essential element of the person-centered approach to counseling. The term refers to the premise that the individual is capable of moving in a self-directive way. Carl Rogers described self-actualization as the individual's "capacity and the tendency...to move forward toward maturity" (Rogers, 1961, p. 35). This move toward maturity enables an individual to move toward self-understanding, growth and change in such a way that his or her life will be enhanced socially, psychologically and spiritually.

Toward an Understanding of Self-actualization

Self-actualization is a process of change. In Rogers' view of self-actualization, a person never reaches a state of being self-actualized, rather, the process of change is an ongoing movement. Being self actualized is a constant experience, not a peak experience. There may be peak experiences whereby the individual is very much in touch with who he or she is as a person, but a person who is not having such an experience is just as self-actualized as the person having a peak experience. In the valley's of one's life, there is self-actualization.

The process of change is maximized through personal relationships, such as therapy in which significant change can take place. While I am convinced that self-actualization takes place all the time, my awareness of that process may be stifled (Bower, 1994). Certain personal relationships open the doors to discovery of the process, though I suspect that discovering the process enhances or facilitates changes (Bozarth, & Brodley, 1986).

The individual makes choices and establishes values differently; he meets frustration with less prolonged physiological tension, he changes in the way he perceives himself and values himself....

The theory of client-centered therapy hypothesizes that the inner changes taking place in therapy will cause the individual after therapy to behave in ways which are less defensive, more socialized, more acceptant of reality in himself and in his social environment and which give evidence of a more socialized system of values. (Rogers, 1961, p. 259)

Self-actualization can also be described as a movement toward newness. There is inherent within the organism a tendency to renew itself on the molecular, biological, psychological and sociological level. This renewal can be seen as a creative movement toward novelty. In this sense, self-actualization is similar to the thinking of philosopher Alfred North Whitehead (1978) concerning "creativity."

"Creativity" is the universal of universals characterizing ultimate matter of fact. It is that ultimate principle by which the many, which are the universe disjunctively, become the one actual occasion, which is the universe conjunctively. It lies in the nature of things that the many enter into complex unity.

"Creativity" is the principle of novelty. An actual occasion is a novel entity diverse from any entity in the "many" which it unifies. Thus "creativity" introduces novelty into the content of the many, which are the universe disjunctively. The "creative advance" is the application of this ultimate principle of Creativity to each novel situation which it originates. (Whitehead, 1978, p. 21)

For Whitehead, the most basic aspect of the universe, the occasion has within it the nature to move in a creative way toward novelty, the ability to add a unique twist to the occasions exists which makes the present occasion different from its predecessors while at the same time incredibly similar to its predecessors. So in each occasion there is the ability to become new. And each occasion has the ability to be influenced by other occasions and to influence other occasions thus creating more novel possibilities and new changes. The movement toward novelty is consistent with Rogers' concept of self-actualization.

Importance of Self-actualization

Although the notion of self-actualization is the very foundation of the person-centered approach, the belief that there exists "in every organism, at whatever level, an underlying flow of movement toward constructive fulfillment of its inherent possibilities" (Rogers, 1977, pp. 7-8) is a not simple concept to appreciate. To do so requires a degree of what Maureen Miller O'Hara has called an "unshakable faith in human beings and their potential" (O'Hara, p. 1). It is essential to have faith in this basic presupposition in order to be person-centered and this is never a simple or easy matter.

A Struggle to Believe

When I first encountered the idea of self-actualization it came into conflict with some of my own presuppositions. The first of these presuppositions was a position which has been assimilated into Christian thought through the centuries: that humankind is sinful by nature. The second presupposition was that human beings are innately self-destructive. The third presupposition was that there exists a destructive tendency in nature which affects humankind. And the fourth presupposition was that I believed that in some individuals self-actualization does not always take place.

The first presupposition that human is sinful by nature has its roots in a rich Christian theological tradition led by such brilliant theologians as St. Augustine, Martin Luther, John Calvin, and John Wesley. This view holds that human beings are totally depraved, alienated, and estranged from God. The cause of this condition is sin, separation from God. Further, sin causes us to remain in rebellion and resistance to God's love and grace. In sin, human beings harm themselves and others.

I agreed wholeheartedly with the New Testament writer, Paul, who said in Romans 6:23a, "The wages of sin is death" (May, & Metzger, 1971). To me death reflected the depth of the sinful human condition. Death was the concrete consequence of the state of being a sinner.

The second presupposition that human beings are innately self-destructive and are damaging to the self is based on our being able to bring harm upon ourselves. We are capable of hurting ourselves, often in relationship with others. We can harm ourselves through misuse of depression, anxiety and a number of other emotions. We can also harm ourselves by psychosomatic and physical means.

My theory about self-destruction was bolstered in my own psychological experience. For me, self-destruction took the form of passive-aggressive, withdrawn behavior, and shyness. Instead of asserting myself in relationships, I would withdraw. Instead of defending my beliefs, I would become frightened and hide. Instead of trusting myself with people, I would become insecure and tentative. Instead of believing in myself, I would fantasize about being successful instead of studying or doing a job well in order to be successful. In this self-destructiveness, I brought suffering upon myself by becoming depressed and anxious. I obsessed about failing to establish solid relations with people. I also failed to meet personal goals. Instead of participating in life, I watched my life go by and I hoped that someone else would take care of me. Self-destruction was/is a real part of my life.

The third presupposition that a destructive tendency exists in nature was based on the hard fact that the world and its people are in turmoil, conflict and chaos. There are all sorts of tragedies and afflictions. War famine, disease and natural disasters are destructive tendencies which are often inflicted upon us by factors within our control. We are too often plagued by these realities.

Finally, the fourth presupposition that in some individuals self-actual-ization does not always take place was based on the perceived difficulty of attaining self-actualization in the real world. Could a person acknowl-edge self-actualization in the patient on the back ward of the psychiatric hospital or in the severely retarded person who cannot even feed himself or herself?

I was bothered that Rogers argued that self-actualization always takes place even in the most difficult of conditions. I thought that for Rogers there was no such thing as self-destructiveness and this seemed naive to me.

Toward Accepting the Concept Self-actualization

In spite of the above barriers, I have come to believe that there is a lot of truth in the concept of self-actualization. As long as a person is alive, there is some capacity for self-direction, even if it is used only for the pur-pose of survival. Self-actualization does always take place on some level. This observation was illustrated by Rogers:

I remember that in my boyhood, the bin in which we stored our win-ter's supply of potatoes was in the basement…The conditions were unfa-vorable, but the potatoes would begin to sprout—pale white sprouts, so unlike the healthy green sprouts they sent up when planted in the soil in the spring. But these sad, spindly sprouts would grow 2 or 3 feet in length as they reached toward the distant light of the window. The sprouts were, in their bizarre, futile growth, a sort of desperate expression of the direc-tional tendency…They would never become plants, never mature, never fulfill their real potential. But under the most adverse circumstances, they were striving to become. Life would not give up, even if it could not flour-ish. In dealing with clients whose lives have been terribly warped, in work-ing with men and women on the back wards of state hospitals, I often think of those potato sprouts. So unfavorable have been the conditions in which these people have developed that their lives often seem abnormal, twisted, scarcely human. Yet, the directional tendency in them can be trusted. The clue to understanding their behavior is that they are striving, in the only ways that they perceive as available to them, to move toward growth, toward becoming. To healthy persons, the results may seem bizarre and futile, but they are life's desperate attempt to become itself. (Rogers 1977, p. 8)

Three factors helped me overcome my initial resistance to Rogers' concept of self-actualization. The first was the use of the word "tendency" in his definition of self-actualization, indicating acknowledgment of impediments to self-actualization. The second factor was the recognition that self-actualization is affected by various elements in a person's life; it does not take place in a vacuum. The third factor was the process of testing Rogers' concept of self-actualization in my own experience.

First, Rogers' use of the word "tendency" seemed to imply acknowledgment a reality of interference with the self-actualization process. He verified this when he wrote, "The actualizing tendency can, of course, be thwarted or warped, but it cannot be destroyed without destroying the organism" (Rogers, 1980, p 118). 1 could accept this notion. There does seem to me to be a destructive tendency which is capable of thwarting the actualization tendency, even to the point of death. However, Rogers trusted that as long as life remains the actualization tendency remains. He insisted that self-actualization can be found even in those so abusively dehumanized, that it appears that nothing of their humanity remains.

In light of these realizations, I began to find a psychological and theological place for the concept of a self-actualizing tendency. If human beings are indeed created in the image of God, all of us must have the ability to move in a self-directive way, a creative way. We have within us the ability to change ourselves; indeed, we cannot keep from changing.

Second, I began to realize that self-actualization is not portrayed as taking place in a vacuum. The process functions at its maximum within a caring environment. Rogers maintained this caring environment can be created by a therapist who is accepting, genuine and empathetic.

I have altered my position slightly. I now believe that self-actualization takes place all the time, but how a it manifests itself within individuals is correlated to a wide variety of factors. If a person deals with a hostile environment at a biological, psychological, or sociological level, he or she will be different than if they deal with a friendly environment. The choices are different on extreme ends of the social spectrum (Bower, 1994).

Third, I began to appreciate the concept of self-actualization through therapeutic experience. I attempted to put Rogers' (1957) "necessary and sufficient conditions" for the therapeutic relationship to the test (Bower, 1985, 1989). I wanted to see if empathy, congruence and unconditional positive regard could indeed be useful in creating an environment which would allow self-actualization to take place with a minimal amount of restriction or inhibition.

A Client and Self-actualization

Near the end of the summer of 1983, 1 began seeing an alcoholic who was not only addicted to alcohol, but also dependent on his wife. His wife was threatening to file for a divorce. It seemed evident that she planned to do so immediately.

Forced from the house by his wife, E moved in with his parents over eighty miles away. He commuted five days a week to work. His work suffered, as he lost four hours out of his working day commuting, in addition to the countless hours he spent drunk.

His previous counselor felt that she could not work with him and referred him to me. His wife degraded and humiliated him, placing on him the entire blame for the break up of the marriage. He accepted that blame and felt guilty and anxious. Of course, with that he drank more. He often stated that he did not know how he would be worth anything as a man without his wife's love. He was anxious about giving her up after fifteen years of marriage.

I tried to utilize the "necessary and sufficient conditions" for therapy. I cannot say I was always successful: at times I experienced impatience and anger with E. As I developed my facility with the person centered approach, I found my feelings of impatience and anger were related to E's impatience and anger, and thus my feelings were valuable clues to his feelings.

As I became better able to be empathic, genuine and accepting, I saw change in E. At first he dreaded living alone from fear of loneliness. He was also afraid of regressing in his addiction to alcohol. After a time, however, E was living alone in his own apartment. He was gainfully employed. He was not taking his ex-wife's accusations and so seriously and belittlement so seriously and he began seeing himself as a person of more worth and value. He had begun not to feel as inferior as he once had. Significant changes had taken place within E because he had the capacity to move toward self-understanding and growth, though these changes had not necessarily come about in a conscious way. I believe that the basic therapeutic conditions of empathy, acceptance and genuineness played a role in facilitating E's changes.

Just a couple of years ago, I heard that E was the director of a substance abuse program though he sent a message to me that he didn't think the non-directive style is helpful for people like him. I beg to differ. He is the evidence for change.

One further illustration of self-actualization.

A baby has fallen out of its walker. There will be a few seconds of feeling painfully the fall. Cries, perhaps wrenching the body, will respond to the painful feelings. But in a few seconds the pain itself will abate. Yet, the sobbing continues. The baby is no longer sobbing in response to the initial fall and hurt; it is now sobbing in response to its own sobbing...It may take several seconds or even minutes for the crying to end. (Jackson, 1981 p. 25)

The sobbing does end. In this illustration comfort was interrupted by a fall on a hard floor. Discomfort prevailed. The baby's falling on the floor caused trauma to skin, tissue and nerves causing pain. Signals were sent to the brain, which in turn sent signals to the voice box and tear glands, making the crying possible.

Eventually, the pain subsided, as did the reaction to the pain. Comfort prevailed. This was not a return to comfort, but a new comfort made possible by the forces present within and about the baby as it reacted to its environment. The baby was exercising the capacity of moving in a self-directive way toward being comfortable. Yet this comfort was obtained in association with the environment within and around the baby.

Presently, I accept the Person-Centered concept of self-actualization. I regard my own life as an example of the self-actualizing tendency. I am no longer the passive-aggressive, shy, and withdrawn person I once was, which gets me into a lot of trouble from time to time. I still struggle with that old personal phenomena. I still struggle with being intimidated by people. However, I have discovered within myself the capacity to understand myself and accept myself and to reach out to meet my needs. I find in this the capacity to be more assertive often over and above my fears.

Since I can see self-actualization in myself, I can recognize it in others. I believe my work with E verifies that fact. A number of other encounters with people have validated self-actualization for me, as well.

Since I believe in the basic presupposition of self-actualization, I have begun developing the concept in a framework which makes sense to me. I find more and more that Rogers's notion of self-actualization provides me with a framework that I can trust.

Summary

Rogers trusted in the self-actualization process. He believed that people can and will move and change in self-directive ways. He believed that if people are given the opportunity, they will become more perceptive of themselves, value themselves more highly and be more accepting.

I have discussed presuppositions which impeded my acceptance of Rogers' concept of self-actualization. I have also discussed ideas which helped me to begin trusting the concept. I believe that the best validation of the idea of self-actualization rests in the changes which occur within individuals. In light of such changes, the concept becomes a reality. Over time, something becomes different about every person. Every person moves in a self-directive way. Every person is self-actualizing.

References

Bower, D. W. (1985). Assumptions and attitudes of the Rogerian person-centered approach to counseling: Implications for pastoral counseling. Unpublished manuscript, Columbia Theological Seminary, Decatur, GA.

Bower, D. W. (1989). **The attributes of five person-centered therapists.** Unpublished doctoral dissertation, University of Georgia, Athens, Ga.

Brodley, B. T., & Bozarth, J. D. (1986). Client-centered psychotherapy: A statement. **The Person-Centered Review, 1,** (3), 262-271.

Jackson, G. E. (1981). **Pastoral care and process theology.** Washington D.C.: University Press of America.

May, H. G., & Metzger, B. M. (1971). **The new Oxford annotated Bible: The Holy Bible: Revised standard version containing the old and new testaments.** New York: Oxford University Press.

O'Hara, M. M. (Date unknown). Person-centered approach as conscientizacao: The works of Carl Rogers and Paul Freire, (Unpublished manuscript).

Rogers, C. R. (1951). **Client-centered therapy.** Boston: Houghton Mifflin.

Rogers, C. R. (1957). The necessary and sufficient conditions of therapeutic personality change. **Journal of Consulting Psychology, 21,** 95-103.

Rogers, C. R. (1961). **On becoming a person.** Boston: Houghton Mifflin.

Rogers, C. R. (1977). **On personal power.** New York: Delta.

Rogers, C. R. (1980). **A way of being.** Boston: Houghton Mifflin.

Whitehead, A. N. (1978). **Process and reality.** New York: The Free Press.

Empathy: The Basic Goal of the Therapist In the Person Centered Approach

Doug Bower

In the Star Trek episode entitled "The Empath," Kirk, Spock and McCoy find themselves kidnaped by two aliens. The only other person initially present is Gem, a beautiful young woman who cannot speak. Kirk and McCoy are taken by the aliens to be experimented upon. Both return with devastating injuries. It is McCoy's injuries which turn out to be the most severe and extensive and brought him near death. Gem is an empath, with the capabilities of curing both men. Kirk's injuries are cured when Gem incorporates and assimilates his injuries into her own body. However, McCoy's injuries have the potential to kill Gem as well. Because of this, she has reluctance about reaching into his world. After agonizing over the danger, Gem agrees to enter McCoy's world and take his injuries into her body. His injuries are cured when Gem overcomes her fear and engages McCoy. Thus both men are healed. Gem survives the encounter but has to be helped by the aliens who had been testing Gem to determine if her planet is worthy enough to be saved from impending destruction of two planets, only one could be saved.

Toward an understanding of empathy

Rogers said that "...it is the counselor's function to assume, in so far as he is able, the internal frame of reference of the client, to perceive the world as the client sees it, to perceive the client himself as he is seen by himself, to lay aside all perceptions from the external frame of reference while doing so, and to communicate something of the empathic understanding to the client" (Rogers, 1951, p. 29). In this way, the therapist assumes the internal frame of reference of the client. hurts and pains are encountered by the therapist.

Empathy is a process, an ongoing encounter between self-actualizing individuals. One person comes, hurt, anguishing, suffering in his or her emotional pain and encounters another person. This other person, the therapist, may be hurting, anguishing, and suffering with emotional of his or her own, but is not using the therapy for working on that discomfort. The therapist engages the client by entering into the client's world as if it were his/her own.

Assuming the World of the Client

The first part of the empathic process involves entering the world of the client. The counselor attempts to this world and interact with it. He or she tries to his world as the client sees it, as much as this possible. "As time has gone by we have come to put increasing stress upon the 'client centeredness' of the relationship, because it is more effective the more completely the counselor concentrates upon trying to understand the client as the client seems to himself" (Rogers, 1951, pp. 420-421).

How can I enter the world of the client? I cannot give up my own existence. I cannot give up my heritage. I cannot give up my mind except through losing consciousness. I have my own being. I cannot become the other person. Can I really begin to gain access to a world of another who has a bank of experiences separate from mine?

It is true that it is impossible to literally enter completely into the world of the client. I cannot know fully the experiences which have been part of producing this other person. It is, however, possible to enter the world of the client in such a way as to be a part of his or her world here and now. The therapist can begin to be a part of that world in the present moment.

Initially, I found the idea of empathy baffling. I could not comprehend the possibility of entering the world of the client. I could comprehend being a part of that world, but I could not think in terms of experiencing the clients feelings and thoughts.

One day, while listening to a tape of a client, I had the important realization that I had been focusing too much on being in the world of the client, at the expense of focusing on entering that world. I imagined coming to someone's house. In order to enter the house I knock on the door. The person may or may not let me in. If I am expected, I am invited in. If I am perceived as trustworthy, I probably will be invited in whether I am expected or not. I enter through the open door. I look around. There are several comfortable places to sit. I sit down. I engage in conversation with my host. I look around the living room. There is a painting on the wall.

"That is an interesting painting."

"My grandfather painted that several years ago," my host says.

I have found out something about my host's world.

"I take it you treasure your grandfather."

"Yes," my host says.

I have discovered something else about his world.

As we talk, I discover more and more about this person's world. His family, his friends, his dog, his in his feelings, and his experiences are all shared in some form. I even find that at times he sweeps dirt under the carpet and stashes junk in the closets. I find that he never washes And there is mildew on the bathroom walls.

I find also that he misses his grandfather. He misses his brothers sisters as well. He longs to visit his parents and friends with whom he grew up. He has a bad kidney and at times has suffered a broken heart.

I have entered a new world. I did not know what I would find. I do not know what else I will learn. It is a separate world which may or may not be similar to my own.

Perceiving the World of the Client

In this phase of perceiving the client's world, it is necessary to experience understanding. The goal for this phase is as Rogers stated:

> ...the therapist is experiencing an accurate, empathic understanding of the client's world as seen from the outside. To sense the client's private world as if it were your own...To sense the client's anger, fear, or confusion...When the client's world is this clear to the therapist, and he moves about in it freely, then he can both communicate his understanding of what is clearly known to the client and can also voice meanings in the client's experience of which the client is scarcely aware. (Rogers, 1961, p. 284)

For Rogers the emphasis was on the perceptions of the client: "...It would appear that for me, as counselor my whole attention and effort upon understanding and perceiving as the client perceives and understands, is a striking operational demonstration of the belief I have in the worth and the significance of this individual client" (Rogers, 1951, p. 35).

In the person-centered approach, there is trust that the client knows a great deal about his world (Bozarth, 1998). The counselor cannot be the expert for the client. The counselor cannot really know what is best for the client. Diagnosis, analysis and interpretations do injustice to the client as they weaken the client's capacity to deal with his own world.

In 1940 1 began to try to change...the politics of therapy. Describing an emerging trend, I said, "This newer approach differs from the older one in that is has a genuinely different goal. It aims directly toward the greater independence and integration of the individual rather than hoping such results will accrue if the counselor assists in solving the problem. The individual and not the problem is the focus...

Therapy is not a matter of doing something to the individual, or of inducing him to so something about himself. It is instead a matter of freeing him for normal growth and development, of removing obstacles so that he can again move forward.

I had described various counseling techniques much in use at that time—such as suggestions, advice, persuasion, and interpretation—and had pointed out that these rested on two basic assumptions: that "the counselor knows best," and that he can find techniques by which to move his client most efficiently to the counselor-chosen goal

I had advanced the view that it was preferable simply to free the client to become an independent, self-directing person

It is obvious that even this premise of client-centered therapy, without going further, has enormous political implications. our educational system, our industrial and military organizations, and many other aspects of our culture take the view that the nature of the individual is such that he cannot be trusted—that he must be guided, instructed, rewarded, punished and controlled by those who are wiser and higher in status. To be sure, we give lip service to a democratic philosophy in which all power is vested in the people, but this philosophy is 'honored more in the breach than in the observance.' Hence simply describing the fundamental premise of client-centered therapy is to make a challenging political statement. (Rogers, 1977, p. 6-9)

In the person-centered approach the counselor through empathy, is able to over come the position of standing over and above the client's world. To be empathic is to trust that what is being shared is a description of the client's world. If the client perceives something, what matters is the client's perception; it is true for the client.

Laying Aside the External Frame of Reference

A goal for the therapist in the person-centered approach is to give up power. Being the expert, telling the client what he or she needs to know, what he or she doesn't know, or what he or she needs to do, violates the approach.

The therapist must lay aside his preoccupation with diagnosis and his diagnostic shrewdness, must discard his tendency to make professional evaluations, must cease his endeavors to formulate an accurate prognosis, must give up the temptation subtly to guide the individual, and must concentrate on one purpose only; that of providing deep understanding and acceptance of the attitudes consciously held at this moment by the client as he explores step by step into the dangerous areas which he has been denying to consciousness. (Rogers, 1951, p. 30)

In therapy, the person-centered therapist can best be empathic by taking the perceptions of the client into the therapist's own world and receiving them with the same integrity as the therapist's own perceptions of experiences. This does not mean the therapist necessarily will suffer as the client suffers, but it does mean taking in the suffering of the client in such a way as to affirm that these hurts are real and genuine perceptions of the client. Part of being empathic means affording the feelings and experiences of the client the same integrity as the therapist's own feelings and experiences. The client's world is just as valid as the therapist's, and the person-centered therapist treats both client's world and the therapist's world with respect.

Communicating Empathic Understanding

A major part of being empathic is the empathic response. Barbara Temaner defines this response this way: "an empathic understanding phrasing can be a restatement, a rephrasing,, a summary or a response which involves elaboration" (Temaner, 1977, p. 6). According to Temaner any other response is subject to distortion by the client or the therapist.

The empathic understanding response or reflection for Temaner means more than some mechanical learned response.

The empathic understanding response is fundamentally a transformation of the client's communication inside the mind and experience of the therapist. A transformation involves a change of form without altering value or meaning. In this context a transformation involves the therapist in taking the meaning of his client's expression into himself and understanding it in the terms of his own covert symbols. On the basis of the transformation the therapist may communicate outwardly, usually with language, in a way that seems likely to communicate to the client. (Temaner, p. 6)

However, reflection has not been universally accepted as the standard tool in therapy. The person-centered theory has been subject to significant criticism concerning the limits of reflection. Reflection seems to have been cast into a stereotype. One person I talked to described an actual interview that therapist he had observed between a person-centered therapist and a client.

Client: I feel very horny.

Therapist: You feel horny.

Client: I think I'll masturbate

Therapist: You think you'll masturbate.

Client: (The patient began masturbating).

I never learned what the therapist did when the client began to masturbate, but observed had the therapist continued to adhere to such a stereotyped version of reflection, he would have masturbated also. This stereotype is a myth.

Jerold Bozarth (1984) argues that reflection as the major empathic response limits the counseling equating of the process of empathy with labeled reflection has resulted in (a) between empathy and reflection, (b) focus on relationship: the mode of empathy conceptual confusion operational methods for acting empathic, and (c) limited empathic response modes of therapists" (p. 59). Bozarth argues that focusing concept of empathy, such that "empathy (even by reflection) is no longer being 'able to adopt his (client's) frame of reference, to perceive with him, yet to perceive with acceptance and respect.' (Rogers, 1951, p.41)." (Bozarth, p. 68). Focusing on a technique distracts from being empathic in that the concentration is on the technique instead of the experience of the client.

Rogers himself felt that reflection and empathy became so mistakenly intertwined that he stopped writing and talking about the two for a number of years:

> …This tendency to focus on the therapist's on the technique of reflection distorts the responses had appalling consequences…The whole approach came, in a few years, to be known as a technique. 'Nondirective therapy,' it was said, 'is the technique of reflecting the client's feelings.' or an even worse caricature was simply that 'in nondirective therapy you repeat the last words the client has said.' I was so shocked by these distortion of our approach that for a number of years I said almost nothing about empathic listening…. (Rogers, 1980, p. 139)

Initially, I found reflection useful myself with person-centered counseling; I still find it useful. My tendency has been to use reflection spontaneously when what the client says is obvious to me. I have also used reflection when I have nothing to say and want to communicate verbally that I am still attending to the client. And I use reflection during times of intense concentration on the client. In these moments of concentration, I find myself saying the same thing the client says. Sometimes I manage to say a word or phrase expressing the client's experience before the client says it. On those occasions, it is almost as if I am the client.

I believe that reflection is far more than repeating the words of the client. It involves sharing in the world of the client. This world includes feelings and thoughts. If there is a world of confusion, the therapist may become confused. If there is joy, the therapist may experience joy. These experiences can be reflections of the client's world.

However, reflection can be misused in various ways. It can, for example, become nothing more than stereotyped repeating of the client's words. Such repetition sounds patronizing and seems to insult the intelligence of the client.

Reflection can also be interruptive of the client (Bower, 1989). Some clients I have heard take time out to verify the reflection for the therapist before they move on. They don't seem to mind the interruptions, but reflections seem to interrupt the direction the client is taking.

In my experience, however, the positive potential of reflection has outweighed the negative possibilities. For me, this realization was supported by a brief encounter I had as a volunteer client with a person-centered therapist. During that encounter, I felt I could say anything I wanted to say. I did not feel threatened in any way. In fact, I was sorry that the brief demonstration was the only encounter I would have with the therapist. I wished her practice were nearby. She utilized reflection in a way that seemed warm and genuine, and I felt understood. She did not just repeat what I said; often she found another word or phrase that captured what I was expressing. She helped me to open doors to new understanding. Yet, I didn't experience her as desiring to open those doors. I thus came to the conclusion that reflection utilized by an empathic person can be a powerful tool for the client's moving toward self-understanding.

A Way Toward Being Empathic

Empathy is a process with several aspects. First, empathy is entering the world of the client. on one occasion I heard a person-centered therapist simply say to the client, "Begin any place you like." I believe that by her words and by her presence in the room she had entered the world of the client. I believe that any comment, statement or question might be what is needed to make an entrance into the client's world. The best way to enter that world might even be silence.

Second, empathy is, in part, perceiving the world of the client from the client's perspective. Asking questions can be one way of perceiving this world. Some time ago I was seeing a client who was separated from his wife. It occurred to me as he talked to ask, "Where is your wife living?" He told me that she was living in a city which was over a hundred miles from where he was living. I found out about his world. There was indeed separation. His wife was not living a few miles away where he might be able to see her. She was living over hundred miles away with her family, who had historically been hostile toward him. Upon further questioning, the client expressed reluctance and fear to travel so far to see his wife only to be attacked verbally and physically by his wife's relatives.

I believe that the primary route toward understanding is listening. When I was beginning my struggle to understand the person-centered approach and to give up my clinical tendency to be confrontive, Jerold Bozarth made one suggestion, one that would prove to be one of the most influential given to me in supervision. "Listen," he said. Not a profound word, but it is a profound action.

Empathy in the person-centered approach also involves laying aside all perceptions from the external frame of reference, and giving up presuppositions about the client. In the person-centered approach the therapist is interested in the perception of the client (Brodley, 1996). Personally, I am more interested in the perceptions of the client as they develop in our relationship. I believe these perceptions and how I am impacted by them can tell me something about the world of the client.

The final aspect of empathy is the communication of being empathic. Communication is a natural part of empathy. Empathy in its purest sense is a form of communication. We often think of communication as being verbal, but it is nonverbal as well. Being empathic carries both the verbal and nonverbal forms of communication. The client, through the verbal and nonverbal communications of the empathic therapist, perceives that he or she is understood.

Summary

This chapter has discussed the process of empathy. The discussion was based on one of Rogers' early articulations of empathy which has been restated and rearticulated by Rogers and others over the years. Empathy is assuming, in so far as is possible, "the internal frame reference of the client, to perceive the world as the client sees it, to perceive the client himself as he is seen by himself, to lay aside all perceptions from the external frame of reference while doing so, and to communicate something of the empathic understanding to the client" (Rogers, 1951, p. 29).

Empathy is the basic goal of the person-centered therapist.

References

Bower, D. W. (1989). **The attributes of five person-centered therapists.** Unpublished doctoral dissertation, University of Georgia, Athens, Ga.

Bozarth, J. D. (1984). Beyond Reflection: Emergent modes of empathy. In R. F. Levant & J. M. Shlien. **Client-centered therapy and the person-centered approach: New directions in theory, research, and practice.** New York: Praeger.

Bozarth, J. D. (1998). Person-centered therapy: A revolutionary paradigm. Ross-on-Rye: PCCS Books.

Brodley, B. T. (1996). Empathic understanding and feelings in client-centered therapy. **The Person-Centered Journal,** 3(1), 22-30.

Rogers, C. R. (1951). **Client-centered therapy.** Boston: Houghton Mifflin.

Rogers, C. R. (1961). **On becoming a person.** Boston: Houghton Mifflin.

Rogers, C. R. (1977). **On personal power.** New York: Delta.

Rogers, C. R. (1980). **A way of being.** Boston: Houghton Mifflin.

Temaner, B. (1977). The empathic understanding response process. Unpublished manuscript.

Acceptance: The Basic Context of the Person-centered Approach

Doug Bower

This chapter presents the basic premises of Rogers' concept of acceptance. It also offers my own views on acceptance, and relates them to a clinical experience.

Acceptance of the client is regarded by Rogers as a major factor in promoting self-actualization. The general word acceptance is used in this chapter to denote this attitudinal- principle that Rogers has referred interchangeably as acceptance, unconditional positive regard and warmth.

One advantage of the use of the word acceptance is that it is more widely understood and less controversial than a term like unconditional positive regard. In fact I some unresolved difficulties with the latter concept myself. I have questions which would preclude my use of the that than have term unconditional positive regard with genuineness and honesty. Some of these difficulties will be discussed later.

In writing about acceptance Rogers said,

To the extent that the therapist finds himself experiencing a warm acceptance of each aspect of the client's experience as being a part of that client, he is experiencing unconditional positive regard...It means that there are no conditions of acceptance, no feeling of "I like you only if you are thus and so." It means a "prizing" of the person, as Dewey used that term. It is at the opposite pole from a selective evaluating attitude—"You are bad in these ways, good in those." It involves as much a feeling of acceptance for the client's expression of negative, "bad," painful, fearful, defensive, abnormal feelings as for his expression of "good," positive, mature, confident, social feelings, as much acceptance of ways in which he is inconsistent as of ways in which he is consistent. It means a caring for the client, but not in a possessive way or in such a way as simply to satisfy the therapist's own needs. It means a caring for the client as a separate person, with permission to have his own feelings, his own experiences. (Rogers, 1957, p. 98)

Acceptance as Warmth

"Can I let myself experience positive attitudes toward this other person—attitudes of warmth, caring, liking, interest, respect?" (Rogers, 1961, p. 52). Feelings of warmth are difficult to articulate. They are better understood by the experience of warmth itself. At best, there seems to be reasons why we say that we have warm feelings toward others. When we feel "good" about another person, we are relaxed. When we are relaxed the blood vessels in our body dilate. There is a relatively unrestricted flow of blood to the hands and feet and other parts of the body . The hands and feet literally become warm. Perhaps this is one reason we describe our vague "positive" feelings toward another person as feelings of warmth.

In therapy this warmth is a feeling of caring for the client. It is a feeling of liking this person who has come for counseling . And it is an interest in the world and perceptions of the client.

Acceptance as Unconditional Positive Regard

Unconditional positive regard refers to the therapist's "willingness for the client to be whatever feeling is going on at that moment—confusion, resentment, fear, anger, courage, love, or pride" (Rogers, 1977, p. 10). The therapist accepts the client, and has warm feelings toward the client. The client has worth to the therapist, and the client is prized. All these attitudes are unconditional. Acceptance is not contingent on the client's being other than he or she already is. The therapist does not accept some of the client's feelings as being valid or appropriate while rejecting others. He or she accepts all that the client is at any given moment during their encounter.

There arises a problem, however: does the therapist accept murder? Is suicide acceptable? Is child molestation or child abuse acceptable? Is theft acceptable? Are antisocial behaviors acceptable? Can I hold in unconditional positive regard the actions of a rapist? In good conscience, I must say that I cannot. This fact, however, does no violence to the concept, because unconditional positive regard has never been intended to refer to specific actions, but rather to persons. I can accept the reality that a child abuser or a rapist or a murderer is a person. He or she may have been an object of abuse or violence as a child. This person well may have grown up subjected to an environment which misdirected his self-actualization. In no way does this force me to condone antisocial, destructive actions.

Another thought is that I, if placed into the same world as the client, might have behaved in similar ways. "There but for the grace of God go I." Where does one cross the fine line to become a murderer, or a child abuser, or a rapist? Where is the fine line between being psychotic and being emotionally "healthy?" The thought of destructive acts sometimes enter the minds of "healthy" individuals. I dare say that most of us at one time or another have come close to being destructive persons.

Do these observations imply that we are not accepting the client if we anticipate destructive behavior and hope that the client can and will stop abusing people or him or herself? If we fail to appreciate the acts of the client are we rejecting him or her? Does acceptance involve placing the client's actions beyond criticism?

Criticism of the person centered-approach often involves these sorts of issues. Critics sometimes cite a joke about a client who jumps out of his therapist's window. The person-centered therapist makes no effort to stop his client. Rogers is reported to have responded, "For the last time, No! I would not let the client jump out the window." Rogers did write though:

Some counselors—usually those with little specific training—have supposed that the counselor's role in carrying on nondirective counseling was merely to be passive and to adopt a laissez faire policy....

This misconception of the approach has led to considerable failure in counseling—and for good reasons. In the first place, the passivity and seeming lack of interest or involvement is experienced by the client as a rejection, since indifference is in no real way the same as acceptance. In the second place, a laissez faire attitude does not in any way indicate to the client that he is regarded as a person of worth. (Rogers, 1951, p. 27)

Perhaps the most accepting, caring, prizing act would be to interfere with the client's intended suicide or murder by calling the police. Perhaps saying to the client, "I don't want you to beat your little boy any more," is a way of expressing warm regard for the client. Such a comment does not imply, "You are the scum of the earth," but rather, "I value you and your child."

Acceptance as unconditional positive regard is nonjudgmental. The therapist is not a judge pronouncing a verdict or condemning the client.

It is impossible to be accurately perceptive of another's inner world if you have formed an evaluative opinion of that person. If you doubt this statement, choose someone you know with whom you deeply disagree and who is, in your judgment, definitely wrong or mistaken. Now try to state that individual's views, beliefs, and feelings so accurately that he or she will agree that you have sensitively and correctly described his or her stance. I predict that nine times out of ten you will fail, because your judgment of the person's views creeps into your description of them. (Rogers 1980, p. 154)

Acceptance is based on the basic trust: that the client can and will move in a self-directive way. This belief in the individual helps make it possible not to be possessive and judgmental.

Writing about tennis, W. Timothy Gallwey addresses the nonjudgmental attitude in terms useable for counseling:

When asked to give up making judgments about one's game the judgmental mind usually protests, "But if I can't hit a backhand inside the court to save my life, do you expect me to ignore my faults and pretend my game is fine? " Be clear about this: letting go of judgments does not mean ignoring errors. It simply means seeing events as they are and not adding anything to them. Nonjudgmental awareness might observe that during a certain match you hit 50 percent of your first serves into the net. It doesn't ignore the fact. It may accurately describe your serve on that day as erratic and seek to discover the causes. Judgment begins when the serve is labeled 'bad' and causes interference with one's playing.... (Gallwey, 1974, p. 36)

Acceptance as Prizing and Worth

Rogers also describes acceptance as prizing. Not only is the client of worth as a person, he or she is desirable to the therapist. The client is special and the therapist maintains a degree of pride in knowing this person. The client is prized though he or she may be a broken, battered and ragged person.

"The primary point of importance here is the attitude held by the counselor toward the worth and the significance of the individual" (Rogers, 1951, p. 20). In the person-centered approach, the counselor comes to view each person as having worth and dignity; the client is valued as a person.

A Hypothesis

Rogers believed that acceptance by the therapist will facilitate self-acceptance in the client. "The message comes through to the recipient that 'this other individual trusts me, thinks I'm worthwhile. Perhaps I am worth something. Perhaps I could value myself. Perhaps I could care for myself" (Rogers, 1980, pp. 152-153) "This acceptance of each fluctuating aspect of this other person makes it for him a relationship of warmth and safety, and the safety of being liked and prized as a person seems a highly important element in a helping relationship" (Rogers, 1961, p. 34).

A Personal Note

As I was beginning to understand the concept of empathy, I started by viewing empathy as the receiving of the client into the therapist's world. As I came to see empathy as Rogers described it, the process of entering the world of the client, I needed a concept to handle the receiving of the client into the therapist's world. Acceptance is that concept. In accepting the client, the therapist opens up his or her world and receives the client.

Through acceptance the client enters the world of the therapist. The client is not there to understand the therapist, but to understand him or herself. The client is there to deal with his or her own problems or desires for growth (whatever growth represents for the client), and he or she is being accepted by the therapist.

The earlier-used image of the home is applicable. No one likes to go to someone's home and be abused or treated disrespectfully. We do not like others to tell us what we are feeling and experiencing, even when their observations are accurate. We might tolerate such behavior, but we do not respect it.

On the other hand, we do like to visit friends who are warm, caring and appreciative; who do not condemn us; who might disagree with us, but who prize us and respect us.

So it is with the client. Rogers argues that a client will treasure and grow from therapy when he or she is accepted. When the therapist receives this person the client will respond to therapy in ways relative to that particular client.

An Illustration

In my own experience as a therapist, I have found acceptance to be a valuable factor in facilitating change in a client. I began seeing a thirty-six year old black woman, S, who had shot and killed her husband after years of abuse. She was tried for murder and found not guilty by reason of self-defense. However, at some point she had developed paranoid beliefs and behaviors. It was not clear whether these tendencies were already in evidence only to be accentuated by the tragic incident, or whether the trauma had initiated her behavior. She was suspicious that people were plotting against her. She heard voices over the intercom at work calling her to have sex with the boss. She talked about her husband as if he were a pimp, and she thought that there were people who wanted to kill her because she had ruined their prostitution ring when she killed her husband. She thought that people on the street were looking at her and that they knew she had killed her husband.

The first thing I did was to accept her, but I found it extremely difficult to enter into and understand her world. It was so garbled and confused that the only understanding I could manage was that it was garbled and confused.

However, I accepted her as paranoid. I liked her. I looked forward to seeing her. I accepted as much of the garbled content of her story, as I could piece together. I accepted her view of her husband as a pimp and whether he really might have been one. I accepted her feeling that people were plotting against her and wondered if indeed someone might be plotting against her. I recalled an old saying that reads "Just because you're paranoid doesn't mean they aren't out to get you."

By the time I terminated my relationship with S, she was more coherent and easier to follow. I found that while her husband was not a pimp, he had slept with a lot of women. I verified that he had abused her. I found that people did reject S because she frightened them with behavior that they regarded as crazy and bizarre. People were afraid she would kill them as well. In fact, in one of her more agitated states, S actually had threatened someone with a gun, in another such state of mind she shot at her brother. There was a lot of reality in S's "craziness." By the time I left the center, S had improved dramatically, though I do not know if she maintained that improvement.

Personally, I do not believe that one hour a week of being empathic was sufficient to bring about the change which took place in this client. Especially in light of the fact that initially I did not understand her world. In this case, I believe that acceptance had more power in respect to change. The acceptance had to start somewhere. Maybe it started with the jury that believed she defended herself and was carried along through the mental center and my counseling/therapy.

A client can take acceptance with him or her. Not only can the client experience acceptance in the counseling relationship, but he or she benefits by knowing that the therapist is willing to continue the acceptance by setting aside another hour. The client can thus take acceptance with him or her through anticipation of the next session, and by remembering that for that period of time, a person was accepting him or unconditionally.

Thus, I believe that my acceptance of S played an important role in facilitating change. S did not become a perfect citizen, but I believe she became a more socially functioning person. I believe with Rogers that acceptance makes a significant impact on the individual. For me, acceptance truly is one of the foundational attitudinal principles for maximizing the self-actualizing tendency.

A Word of Caution

I do not believe that it is possible always to be accepting of the client during each moment of therapy; neither does Rogers. A footnote in his article on the "Necessary and Sufficient Conditions…(Rogers, 1957) reveals this:

The phrase "unconditional positive regard" may be an unfortunate one, since it sounds like an absolute, an all or nothing dispositional concept. It is probably evident from the description that completely unconditional positive regard would never exist except in theory. From a clinical and experiential point of view I believe that the most accurate statement is that the effective therapist experiences unconditional positive regard for the client during many moments of this contact with him, yet from time to time he experiences only a conditional positive regard—and perhaps at times a negative regard, though this is not likely in effective therapy. It is in this sense that unconditional positive regard exists as a matter of degree in any relationship." (p. 98)

If I have a client whom I cannot accept unconditionally, if extreme bias, if hard feelings, or other factors block acceptance, I can refer the client to a colleague. Fortunately, I have yet to have this experience.

Summary

I believe the word acceptance is the most appropriate word for this second attitudinal principle. I have chosen it because I believe that it is broad enough to include warmth, prizing, and unconditional positive regard, with all their different connotations.

It is the torn and broken person whom the therapist accepts. It is the person who has lost something. It is the person who appears to be falling apart who is accepted. Often the person coming for therapy is being rejected for not being a "together" person. The client's friends and relatives may cry, "Make him into something new." The therapist accepts and prizes this person. To the therapist, the client is special for being what he or she is, a person with tremendous capabilities as well as very real limitations.

Acceptance is of major importance in maximizing the self-actualization process. Yet, even though my client, S, seemed to benefit most because of my initial acceptance of her, I contend that in most cases acceptance, without the empathy and congruence of the therapist, is not sufficient in itself.

References

Gallwey, W. T. (1974). **The inner game of tennis**. New York: Random House

Rogers, C. R. (1951). **Client-centered therapy**. Boston: Houghton Mifflin

Rogers, C. R. (1957). The necessary and sufficient conditions of therapeutic personality change. **Journal of Consulting Psychology**, 21, 95-103.

Rogers, C. R. (1961). **On becoming a person**. Boston: Houghton Mifflin.

Rogers, C. R. (1977). **On personal power**. New York: Delta.

Rogers, C. R. (1980). A **way of Being**. Boston: Houghton Mifflin

Congruence: The Basic State
of the Therapist In the
Person-Centered Approach

Doug Bower

Until now this study has focused on the therapist's view of the client. This chapter will examine the basic state of the therapist, including the therapist's own way of being and the therapist's experiences of him or herself in relation to the client.

Initially, I was concerned that the person-centered therapist might be minimized to the point of losing him or herself during therapy. I was afraid that the therapist's own feelings, thoughts and experiences would be overlooked. This chapter acknowledges the person of the therapist be dealing with the Rogerian concept of congruence.

A Definition of Congruence

Congruence has been defined as "the quality or state of agreeing or coinciding." The related word, congruous, is defined as "being in agreement, harmony, or correspondence." "To come together," is the idea.

Rogers described congruence as follows:

The more the therapist is herself in the relationship, putting up no professional front or personal facade, the greater is the likelihood that the client will change and grow in a constructive manner. It means that the therapist is openly being the feelings and attitudes that are flowing within

at the moment. The term transparent catches the flavor of this element—
the therapist makes herself transparent to the client; the client can see
right through what the therapist is in the relationship; the client experiences no holding back on the part of the therapist. As for the therapist,
what she is experiencing is available to awareness, can be lived in the relationship, and be communicated if appropriate. Thus there is a close
matching, or congruence, between what is being experienced at the gut
level, what is present in awareness, and what is expressed to the client.
(Rogers, 1977, p. 9)

The State of Being Congruent

Two terms that are essential to Rogers' view of congruence are "self"
and "self concept."

Self

Self can be described as an individual's [personal] self-experience which
is "any event or entity in the phenomenal field discriminated by the individual which is also discriminated as 'self,' 'me,' 'I,' or related thereto"
(Rogers 1959, p. 200). The self is the actual experience of the person,
including thoughts and emotions. The self is comprised of the total experiences of the person.

Somatic experiences are an important part of this total. All somatic
functions contribute to the formulation and maintenance of the self, and
if one's physiology is altered, the self is altered.

Another aspect important to the self is the social environment. The
social environment is influential on the self which is not possible without
an environment. The people a person encounters play a part in the formulation of the self. The social does not formulate the self; the self is actualized only by its self. However, as the social environmental changes, the
self is impacted by these changes. Thus, the loss of a loved one or a major
move can and will play a part in changing the self as the self adjusts to a
new set of events and experiences.

The mental or psychological is another component of the self. This aspect includes the physiology of the brain, without which there would be no mental or psychological functioning, no discrimination process regarding the events or entities in the person's phenomenal field, no thought processes, and no emotional processes. The mental component would is the most crucial to Rogers' idea of self.

Self Concept

The self concept is "the organized, consistent conceptual gestalt composed of perceptions of the characteristics of the 'I' or 'me' and the perceptions of the relationships of the 'I' or 'me' to others and to various aspects of life, together with the values attached to these perceptions" (Rogers, 1959, p. 200). The self concept is that which the person perceives him or herself to be. This perception is influenced by others' perceptions of the person, sometimes to the extent that the person becomes the person of those perceptions. In this case he or she denies his or her own self. In any case, the self concept is the self as perceived.

Incongruence a Key to Congruence

A key to understanding congruence in the therapist is Rogers' definition of incongruence. Incongruence is a discrepancy…between the self as perceived, and the actual experience of the organism. Thus the individual may perceive himself as having characteristics a, b, and c, and experiencing feelings x, y, and z. An accurate symbolization of his experience would, however, indicate 4 characteristics c, d, and e, and feelings v, w, x. (Rogers, 1959, p. 203)

When a person is incongruent, there is a difference between the experiences which comprise the actual self and the perceptions of those self experiences. The experiences are blocked from awareness. Rogers says that this state creates problems "of tension and internal confusion" (Rogers, 1959, p. 203).

The Congruent Therapist

When the therapist is congruent there is no discrepancy between the self and the self concept, at least during the time of therapeutic interaction. The two, self and self concept, are in relative harmony or agreement.

Rogers does not view being congruent as being a constant state for any therapist or any person. He argues that inasmuch as the therapist is congruent in the therapeutic situation, growth can take place within the client. The self-actualization process, the process of perceiving the self in relationship to its real experiences, can be maximized in relationship with a congruent therapist.

It is only by providing the genuine reality which is in me, that the other person can successfully seek for the reality in him. I have found this to be true even when the attitudes I feel are not attitudes with which I am pleased, or attitudes which seem conducive to a good relationship. It seems extremely important to be real. (Rogers, 1961, p. 33)

The Congruent Relationship

A second aspect of congruence is evidenced in the coming together of the therapist and the client. Until the therapist is congruent with him or herself, he or she cannot be empathic with another. Since empathy is the process of entering the world of the client, it is a coming together of a client and a therapist. In essence, empathy is the therapist's becoming congruent, as much as possible, with the client. In the person-centered approach, the therapist who is congruent can then be congruent with another. The therapist can thus let the client be him or herself.

The Therapist as Real and Genuine

The congruent therapist accepts his own thoughts feelings, and experiences. He/she is real. He/she is genuine. He/she experiences anger, sexual urges, depression, joy, love, and hate. Being aware of these experiences, the congruent therapist can accept these as being a significant part of his or her self. It is the denial of one's experiences which is the basis for incongruence.

The therapist who can accept him or herself and his or her experiences can accept these same kinds of experiences as being a part of others. This acceptance makes it possible to be congruent with the client. The therapist who can empathize, being secure enough with his or her own world, is not overwhelmed by the feelings, thoughts and being of the client's world and he or she can thus become empathically one with the client.

The client can perceive the congruent therapist as being genuine and real. The client experiences the therapist for what he is.

Each of us knows individuals whom we somehow trust because we sense they are being what they are, that we are dealing with the person himself, not with a polite or professional front. It is this quality of congruence which we sense which research has found to be associated with successful therapy. (Rogers, 1961, p. 61)

Rogers makes this genuineness sound almost mystical when referring to "individuals whom we somehow trust" because we somehow we mysteriously sense this genuineness. I do not believe that it is a matter of mystery. Genuineness can be communicated both verbally and nonverbally. The feelings the therapist is experiencing are available to him, available to his awareness, and he is able to live these feelings, be them, and able to communicate them if appropriate."(Rogers, 1961, p. 61)

A Missing Dimension

Tapes by person-centered therapists, reveal that the therapists do not share their own experiences with their clients (Bower, 1986). Often disclosure seems to go no further than an occasional admission that the therapist is having difficulty comprehending what client has said. It seems not to be a general practice for the therapist to communicate his or her own inner experiences to the client. The tendency seems to be to reflect the client's perception without sharing the inner impact that the client has had on the therapist.

However, Rogers is willing to share himself with his clients. In the "Gloria" film, he said, "I think you'd make a pretty nice daughter." In a film illustrating his group theory, he wiped tears from his eyes when interacting with a young woman. In writing about confrontation, Rogers demonstrates this further:

I tend to confront individuals on specifics of their behavior. "I don't like the way you chatter on. Seems to me you give each message three of four times. I wish you would stop when you've completed your message." "To me you seem sort of like silly putty. Someone seems to reach you, to make a dent in you, but then it all springs back into place as though you hadn't been touched."

And I like to confront another person only with feelings I am willing to claim as my own. These may at times be very strong. "Never in my life have I been so pissed off at a group as I am at this one." Or, to one man in the group, "I woke up this morning feeling, 'I never want to see you again.'"

To attack a person's defenses seems to me judgmental. If one says, "You're hiding a lot of hostility," or "You are being highly intellectual probably because you are afraid of your own-feelings," I believe such judgments and diagnoses are the opposite of facilitative. If, however, what I perceive as the person's coldness frustrates me or his intellectualizing irritates me, or his brutality to another person angers me, then I would like to face him with the frustration or the irritation or the anger that exists in me. To me this is very important. (Rogers, 1970, pp. 58-59)

This approach is very open, genuine and real. I know what is happening with the therapist. The real and genuine therapist can and will have feelings during therapy, as the client's world makes an impact on the therapist's world. There will be feelings present', and not always pleasant ones. There can be experiences of fatigue or feelings of impatience. However, it does not seem to be a pattern for person-centered therapists to verbally claim these experiences during therapy, in spite of the theoretical and practical example of Rogers himself.

The experiences of the therapist can be the basis of valuable empathic responses. Bozarth (1984) argues for attending to oneself during therapy as well as attending to the client. The reason for this is that what the therapist experiences during therapy can be related to the experiences of the client. One of my clients began sessions with "I don't have anything to talk about." I tended to feel uncomfortable during the beginning of the sessions. "What are we going to do this hour?" I wondered. I would think that my thoughts and feelings of boredom could have been utilized in an empathic encounter, but unfortunately, I did not check my experiences out with the client. Thus, I remain to this day unable to confirm my suspicion. However, in another client, I encountered a very hostile and agitated person. I experienced feelings of anger, hostility and agitation. I also experienced fear. I now believe that my experiences were related to the experiences of the client.

Implications

I believe that Rogers's concepts about genuineness and transparency can open doors to communication therapy. I cannot, however, believe that it is possible always to be empathic and accepting of a client. It seems to be a facade to take the role of the stereotypical person-centered therapist. To be real might mean saying to the client, "I don't understand what you are saying." Or, "I am feeling very angry right now." Or, "I am beginning to feel like I am being manipulated." I do not believe that these examples violate the principle or intention of Rogers' theory: they may very well be appropriate genuine responses.

I believe the excessive use of reflection can handicap the communication of the therapist. The client does not know what the therapist feels, thinks or experiences. In reflection, the client encounters only the reflection of him or herself and not his or her impact on another person. For instance, a person's behavior might stimulate irritation in others. With the exclusive use of reflection, the client might never know that his or her behavior is met with irritation by others or the therapist.

I believe that the concept of congruence holds tremendous potential for dealing with major problems with clients. "I like you and I don't want to see you go to jail for murder," is a real and genuine response. "I'd miss you and it would hurt to know that you killed yourself," is also genuine and real.

I believe that a great deal of criticism of the person-centered approach can be averted by allowing the therapist to be him or herself, instead of insisting that he or she become exclusively reflective and thus limited to a stereotypical approximation of empathy.

Summary

Rogers' notion of congruence has two aspect: a coming together of the therapist's self and the self concept, and the subsequent ability for the therapist to enter into the world of the client, genuinely accept the client and be viewed as being real by the client.

The therapist has a wealth of experiences during therapy. These experiences may be related to the experiences of the client, and thus, they can be utilized to help the therapist understand the inner world of the client.

What has impressed me about the person-centered theory are the many different ways of being congruent and genuine (Bower, 1985, 1989). They appear in the multitude of manifestations of the expression of empathy, acceptance and congruence. These possible expressions need to be explored, to expand the repertoire of presently reflective and empathic responses available to the therapist.

References

Bower, D. W. (1985). Assumptions and attitudes of the Rogerian person-centered approach to counseling: Implications for pastoral counseling. Unpublished manuscript, Columbia Theological Seminary, Decatur, GA.

Bower, D. W. (1989). **The attributes of five person-centered therapists.** Unpublished doctoral dissertation, University of Georgia, Athens, Ga.

Bozarth, J. D. (1984). Beyond Reflection: Emergent modes of empathy. In R. F. Levant & J. M. Shlien. **Client-centered therapy and the person-centered approach: New directions in theory, research, and practice.** New York: Praeger.

Rogers, C. R. (1959). A theory of therapy, personality, and interpersonal relationships, as-developed in the client-centered framework. In **Psychology: A study of science,** Vol III: **Formulations of the person and the social context,** S. Koch (Ed.) New York: McGraw-Hill

Rogers, C. R. (1961). **On becoming a person.** Boston: Houghton Mifflin.

Rogers, C. R. (1970). **On encounter groups.** New York: Perennial Library.

Rogers, C. R. (1977). **On personal power.** New York: Delta.

About the Author

Doug Bower is a licensed professional counselor, a circuit rider with the North Georgia Conference of the United Methodist Church, and a registered nurse. He offers counseling through Counseling Ministries, rides the Bishop Circuit, and volunteers his limited nursing services as a sports medicine consultant to a local high school football team in Athens, Georgia. In addition he is an adjunct faculty member in the counseling psychology department at Ft. Valley State University in Ft. Valley, Georgia.

Doug was introduced to the person-centered approach in seminary, but did not feel he appreciated the approach until he studied with Jerold Bozarth at the University of Georgia beginning in 1982. Since then he has helped organize and participated in every Warm Springs Person-Centered Workshop since it was founded by Jerold Bozarth in 1987. He has been a reviewer, assistant editor, and managing editor for the Person-Centered Journal. He also was the publisher and editor for the Person-Centered Periodical. He has written a handful of articles pertaining to various aspects of the person-centered approach, and has presented at person-centered workshops.